Neurocritical Care

Editor

CHERYLEE W.J. CHANG

CRITICAL CARE CLINICS

www.criticalcare.theclinics.com

Consulting Editor
RICHARD W. CARLSON

October 2014 • Volume 30 • Number 4

ELSEVIER

1600 John F. Kennedy Boulevard • Suite 1800 • Philadelphia, Pennsylvania, 19103-2899

http://www.theclinics.com

CRITICAL CARE CLINICS Volume 30, Number 4
October 2014 ISSN 0749-0704, ISBN-13: 978-0-323-32603-2

Editor: Patrick Manley
Developmental Editor: Casey Jackson

Critical Care Clinics (ISSN: 0749-0704) is published quarterly by Elsevier Inc., 360 Park Avenue South, New York, NY 10010-1710. Months of issue are January, April, July, and October. Business and Editorial Offices: 1600 John F. Kennedy Blvd., Suite 1800, Philadelphia, PA 19103-2899. Customer Service Office: 6277 Sea Harbor Drive, Orlando, FL 32887-4800. Periodicals postage paid at New York, NY and additional mailing offices. Subscription prices are $210.00 per year for US individuals, $503.00 per year for US institution, $100.00 per year for US students and residents, $255.00 per year for Canadian individuals, $630.00 per year for Canadian institutions, $300.00 per year for international individuals, $630.00 per year for international institutions and $150.00 per year for Canadian and foreign students/residents. To receive student/resident rate, orders must be accompanied by name of affiliated institution, date of term, and the signature of program/residency coordinator on institution letterhead. Orders will be billed at individual rate until proof of status is received. Foreign air speed delivery is included in all *Clinics* subscription prices. All prices are subject to change without notice. POSTMASTER: Send address changes to *Critical Care Clinics*, Elsevier Periodicals Customer Service, 11830 Westline Industrial Drive, St. Louis, MO 63146. **Customer Service: 1-800-654-2452 (US). From outside of the US, call 1-314-447-8871. Fax: 1-314-447-8029. E-mail: journalscustomerservice-usa@elsevier.com (for print support) or journalsonlinesupport-usa@elsevier.com (for online support).**

Reprints. For copies of 100 or more of articles in this publication, please contact the Commercial Reprints Department, Elsevier Inc., 360 Park Avenue South, New York, NY 10010-1710. Tel.: 212-633-3874; Fax: 212-633-3820; E-mail: reprints@elsevier.com.

Critical Care Clinics is also published in Spanish by Editorial Inter-Medica, Junin 917, 1er A, 1113, Buenos Aires, Argentina.

Critical Care Clinics is covered in *MEDLINE/PubMed (Index Medicus), EMBASE/Excerpta Medica, Current Concepts/ Clinical Medicine, ISI/BIOMED,* and *Chemical Abstracts*.

Contributors

CONSULTING EDITOR

RICHARD W. CARLSON, MD, PhD
Chairman Emeritus, Director, Medical Intensive Care Unit, Department of Medicine, Maricopa Medical Center; Professor, University of Arizona College of Medicine; Professor, Department of Medicine, Mayo Graduate School of Medicine, Phoenix, Arizona

EDITOR

CHERYLEE W.J. CHANG, MD, FACP, FCCM
Past President, Neurocritical Care Society; Medical Director, Neuroscience Institute/ Neurocritical Care; Director, Stroke Center, The Queen's Medical Center; Associate Clinical Professor of Medicine and Surgery, John A. Burns School of Medicine, University of Hawaii, Honolulu, Hawaii

AUTHORS

FAWAZ AL-MUFTI, MD
Columbia University College of Physicians and Surgeons, New York, New York

THOMAS BLECK, MD, FCCM
Departments of Neurological Sciences, Neurosurgery, Anesthesiology and Internal Medicine, Rush University Medical Center, Chicago, Illinois

GRETCHEN M. BROPHY, PharmD, BCPS, FCCP, FCCM
Professor, Departments of Pharmacotherapy & Outcomes Science and Neurosurgery, Medical College of Virginia Campus, Virginia Commonwealth University, Richmond, Virginia

SHEILA CHAN, MD
Neurocritical Care Program, Department of Neurology, University of California, San Francisco, San Francisco, California

JAN CLAASSEN, MD, PhD, FNCS
Assistant Professor of Neurology and Neurosurgery; Head of Neurocritical Care; Medical Director of the Neurological Intensive Care Unit, Columbia University College of Physicians and Surgeons, New York, New York

MICHAEL N. DIRINGER, MD
Neurocritical Care Section, Department of Neurology, Washington University School of Medicine, St. Louis, Missouri

DAVID M. GREER, MD, MA, FCCM, FAHA, FNCS
Department of Neurology, Yale University School of Medicine, New Haven, Connecticut

J. CLAUDE HEMPHILL III, MD, MAS
Neurocritical Care Program, Department of Neurology, Brain and Spinal Injury Center, San Francisco General Hospital, University of California, San Francisco; Professor of Neurology and Neurological Surgery, Department of Neurological Surgery, University of California, San Francisco, San Francisco, California

THERESA HUMAN, PharmD, BCPS
Neuroscience Clinical Specialist, Barnes-Jewish Hospital, Washington University in St. Louis, St. Louis, Missouri

SYED O. KAZMI, MD
Division of Vascular Neurology and Neurocritical Care, Department of Neurology, Baylor College of Medicine, Houston, Texas

MATTHEW A. KOENIG, MD, FNCS
Associate Medical Director of Neurocritical Care, Neuroscience Institute, The Queen's Medical Center; Assistant Professor of Medicine, The University of Hawaii John A. Burns School of Medicine, Honolulu, Hawaii

GEORGIA KORBAKIS, MD
Department of Neurological Sciences, Rush University Medical Center, Chicago, Illinois

JUAN ANTONIO LLOMPART-POU, MD, PhD
Intensive Care Department, Son Espases Hospital, Palma de Mallorca, Balearic Islands, Spain

NELSON J. MALDONADO, MD
Division of Vascular Neurology and Neurocritical Care, Department of Neurology, Baylor College of Medicine, Houston, Texas

EDWARD MANNO, MD
Neurological Institute, Cleveland Clinic Foundation, Cleveland, Ohio

KRISTINE H. O'PHELAN, MD
Department of Neurology, University of Miami-Miller School of Medicine, Miami, Florida

JULES OSIAS, MD, MPH
Neurological Institute, Cleveland Clinic Foundation, Cleveland, Ohio

JON PEREZ-BARCENA, MD, PhD
Department of Neurology, University of Miami-Miller School of Medicine, Miami, Florida

AMANDA K. RAYA, MD
Neurocritical Care Section, Department of Neurology, Washington University School of Medicine, St. Louis, Missouri

JOSE IGNACIO SUAREZ, MD
Professor of Neurology; Head, Division of Vascular Neurology and Neurocritical Care, Department of Neurology, Baylor College of Medicine, Houston, Texas

STACY A. VOILS, PharmD, MS, BCPS
Clinical Assistant Professor, Department of Pharmacotherapy and Translational Research, University of Florida College of Pharmacy, Gainesville, Florida

TEDDY S. YOUN, MD
Neurocritical Care Fellow, Division of Neurocritical Care and Emergency Neurology, Department of Neurology, Yale University School of Medicine, New Haven, Connecticut

Contents

> Although neurocritical care as a subspecialty is a relatively young field of medicine, its origins can be traced back to ancient times. This article focuses on the progression of neurocritical care from prehistoric trepanation procedures, through the development of mechanical ventilation, management of increased intracranial pressure, and traumatic brain injury, to the establishment of the first "real" intensive care units, and finally to modern monitoring in neurocritical care, management of post-cardiac arrest patients, and the diagnosis of brain death. This article also focuses on the future direction of neurocritical care.

> Acute ischemic stroke is the fourth leading cause of death and the leading cause of disability in the United States. Stroke is a medical emergency. The development of stroke systems of care has changed the way practitioners view and treat this devastating disease. Ample evidence has shown that patients presenting early and receiving intravenous thrombolytic therapy have the best chance for significant improvement in functional outcome, particularly if they are transported to specialized stroke centers. Early detection and management of medical and neurologic complications is key at preventing further brain damage in patients with acute ischemic stroke.

> Primary, spontaneous intracerebral hemorrhage (ICH) confers significant early mortality and long-term morbidity worldwide. Advances in acute care including investigative, diagnostic, and management strategies are important to improving outcomes for patients with ICH. Physicians caring for patients with ICH should anticipate the need for emergent blood pressure reduction, coagulopathy reversal, cerebral edema management, and surgical interventions including ventriculostomy and hematoma evacuation. This article reviews the pathogenesis and diagnosis of ICH, and details the acute management of spontaneous ICH in the critical care setting according to existing evidence and published guidelines.

> Nontraumatic subarachnoid hemorrhage from intracranial aneurysm rupture presents with sudden severe headache. Initial treatment focuses on airway management, blood pressure control, and extraventricular drain for hydrocephalus. After identifying the aneurysm, they may be clipped surgically or endovascularly coiled. Nimodipine is administered to maintain a euvolemic state and prevent delayed cerebral ischemia (DCI). Patients may receive anticonvulsants. Monitoring includes serial neurologic assessments, transcranial Doppler ultrasonography, computed tomography perfusion, and angiographic studies. Treatment includes augmentation of blood pressure and cardiac output, cerebral angioplasty, and intra-arterial infusions of vasodilators. Although early mortality is high, about one-half of survivors recover with little disability.

> Intracranial pressure (ICP) monitoring is considered the standard of care in the majority of neurosurgical centers in North America and Europe. ICP is a reflection of the relationship between alterations in craniospinal volume and the ability of the craniospinal axis to accommodate added volume. ICP cannot be reliably estimated from any specific clinical feature or CT finding and must be directly measured. This review describes methods of monitoring ICP and how monitoring technique can provide additional information and provides key points regarding the treatment of intracranial hypertension in the neuro-ICU.

> Status epilepticus (SE) is a life-threatening medical and neurologic emergency requiring prompt recognition and treatment. SE may be classified into convulsive and nonconvulsive, based on the presence of rhythmic jerking of the extremities. Refractory status epilepticus is defined as ongoing seizures failing to respond to first- and second-line anticonvulsant drug therapy and carries a high morbidity and mortality. Treatment efficacy, morbidity, and mortality are directly related to delays in starting therapy. Benzodiazepines are first-line therapy, usually followed by phenytoin/fosphenytoin or valropoic acid. A low threshold should exist for obtaining an urgent electroencephalogram.

> Brain injury represents the major cause of long-term disability and mortality among patients resuscitated from cardiac arrest. Brain-directed therapies include maintenance of normal oxygenation, hemodynamic support to optimize cerebral perfusion, glycemic control, and targeted temperature management. Pertinent guidelines and recommendations are reviewed for brain-directed treatment. The latest clinical trial data regarding targeted temperature management are also reviewed. Contemporary

prognostication among initially comatose cardiac arrest survivors uses a combination of clinical and electrophysiologic tests. The most recent guidelines for prognostication after cardiac arrest are reviewed. Ongoing research regarding the effects of induced hypothermia on prognostic algorithms is also reviewed.

Neuromuscular sequelae are common in the critically ill. Critical illness polyneuropathy and critical illness myopathy are neuromuscular complications of sepsis or iatrogenic complications of treatments required in intensive care. This article discusses the diagnosis, treatment, and prognosis of these disorders based on a literature review. This review found that glycemic control, early mobilization, and judicious use of steroids and neuromuscular blocking agents are the primary approaches to reduce the incidence and severity of neuromuscular complications in affected patients.

Adverse drug effects often complicate the care of critically ill patients. Therefore, each patient's medical history, maintenance medication, and new therapies administered in the intensive care unit must be evaluated to prevent unwanted neurologic adverse effects. Optimization of pharmacotherapy in critically ill patients can be achieved by considering the need to reinitiate home medications, and avoiding drugs that can decrease the seizure threshold, increase sedation and cognitive deficits, induce delirium, increase intracranial pressure, or induce fever. Avoiding medication-induced neurologic adverse effects is essential in critically ill patients, especially those with neurologic injury.

The concept of brain death developed with the advent of mechanical ventilation, and guidelines for determining brain death have been refined over time. Organ donation after brain death is a common source of transplant organs in Western countries. Early identification and notification of organ procurement organizations are essential. Management of potential organ donors must take into consideration specific pathophysiologic changes for medical optimization. Future aims in intensive and neurocritical care medicine must include reducing practice variability in the operational guidelines for brain death determination, as well as improving communication with families about the process of determining brain death.

CRITICAL CARE CLINICS

ISSUE OF RELATED INTEREST

Neurosurgery Clinics, July 2013 (Vol. 24, No. 3)
Neurocritical Care in Neurosurgery
Paul A. Nyquist, Marek A. Mirski, and Rafael J. Tamargo, *Editors*
Available at: http://www.neurosurgery.theclinics.com/

**DOWNLOAD
Free App!**

Review Articles
THE CLINICS

NOW AVAILABLE FOR YOUR iPhone and iPad

Preface

The Discovery, Recognition, and Rebirth of a Specialty

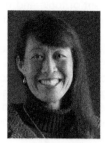

Cherylee W.J. Chang, MD, FACP, FCCM
Editor

As you will read in the introductory chapter of the Evolution of Neurocritical Care, acute neurologic surgical procedures have been documented as early as 10,000 BC through findings of trephined skulls; however, the recognition of modern acute care neurology has been much more recent.

Acute life-threatening neuromuscular respiratory failure that occurred during the polio epidemics in the 1940s and 1950s fueled the need for adequate mechanical ventilation for patient survival. Although these systemic complications were caused by a neurologic entity, the mantle of intensive care for these patients was thereafter assumed by pulmonologists and anesthesiologists. During the next few decades, in the critical care arena, neurologists for the most part were relegated to a diagnostician role until pioneers such as Werner Hacke, Allan Ropper, Daniel Hanley, Matthew Fink, Cecil Borel, and Thomas Bleck took the lead in creating subspecialized neurocritical units dedicated to not only neurosurgical patients but also patients with other neurologic illnesses. These forward-thinking individuals founded robust neurocritical care training programs through which nearly every practitioner of neurocritical care has their educational roots.

The advent of acute thrombolysis for ischemic stroke changed the landscape for acute stroke care. No longer are neurologic patients placed in the furthest reaches of the emergency department where the best advice was to administer an aspirin and call the neurologist in the morning. Now we know indeed that time lost is brain lost at the estimated cost of 1.9 million neurons each minute. Acute stroke care helped bring neurologists back into the fold of critical care neurology and in this area there is much to do and learn.

Not only are treatment advances occurring in acute stroke alone but also recent understanding of receptors and ion channels on excitatory and inhibitory synapses has led to a doubling of approved anticonvulsant medications with novel mechanisms of

Crit Care Clin 30 (2014) ix–x
http://dx.doi.org/10.1016/j.ccc.2014.07.001
0749-0704/14/$ – see front matter © 2014 Elsevier Inc. All rights reserved.

criticalcare.theclinics.com

action in the last 15 years. Renewing old concepts of neuroprotection by hypothermia has revitalized the use of acute temperature regulation following cardiac arrest for improved neurologic outcomes. Studies are ongoing to find acute treatment of traumatic brain injury (TBI) and acute spinal cord injury. Rapid care has become the hallmark for patients suffering TBI, status epilepticus, stroke, subarachnoid hemorrhage, and with hypoxic ischemic brain injury. Acute treatment and enhanced care in the neurointensive care unit now require the development of tools and methods for neurologic prognostication and the evaluation and management of brain-dead patients.

It is inspiring that multidisciplinary practitioners, hospitals, training programs, other medical and surgical specialties, and their national and international societies have come to recognize and embrace the neurologic subspecialty of neurocritical care. The Neurocritical Care Society, established in 2003, has grown from 70 members to over 1400 members in 2014. Other societies of critical care experts are incorporating topics related to neurologic illness in the ICU into their annual meetings to meet the growing recognition and desire for more education in this blossoming field.

I hope that you will enjoy this issue of *Critical Care Clinics*. It is my privilege to showcase my esteemed colleagues; they are experts who have integrated into their articles the international work done in TBI, stroke, intracerebral hemorrhage, therapeutic hypothermia, status epilepticus, subarachnoid hemorrhage, intracranial pressure management, neuropharmacology, neuromuscular ICU complications, and brain death.

This issue of *Critical Care Clinics* is dedicated to my QET4D colleagues and all the forward-thinking practitioners of all specialties and disciplines in neurocritical care for their tireless hard-work and dedication that they give their patients. I especially would like to thank my mentors, Thomas Bleck, Jonathon Truwit, and Stephen Wasserman, who helped support my pursuit of a career in neurocritical care before nearly any one else recognized this budding subspecialty. My appreciation goes to Art Ushijima and Darlena Chadwick, who, as hospital administrators for The Queen's Medical Center, have unflaggingly supported the mission of neurocritical care expertise for the State of Hawaii. My thanks to my parents, Tom and Jane, and especially to my children, Christina and Scott Meyer, for their love and understanding when I was working in the ICU. Despite awareness of the sacrifices a family makes in service to others, I am grateful that they see the sacrifices are worthwhile, such that they have integrated into their lives the mission to serve others, to prevent injury and disease, improve survival, and make lives better.

Cherylee W.J. Chang, MD, FACP, FCCM
Neuroscience Institute/Neurocritical Care
Stroke Center
The Queen's Medical Center
John A. Burns School of Medicine, University of Hawaii
1301 Punchbowl Street, QET5
Honolulu, HI 96813, USA

E-mail address:
cchang@queens.org

Erratum

Errors were made in the April 2014 issue (Volume 30, number 2) of *Critical Care Clinics* regarding the exclusion of two authors from the title page of the article "Advanced Ultrasound Procedures." On page 305, the complete list of authors should read as follows: Nicholas Hatch, Teresa S. Wu, Laurel Barr, and Pedro J. Roque.

Crit Care Clin 30 (2014) xi
http://dx.doi.org/10.1016/j.ccc.2014.07.002
0749-0704/14/$ – see front matter © 2014 Elsevier Inc. All rights reserved.

criticalcare.theclinics.com

The Evolution of Neurocritical Care

Georgia Korbakis, MD[a],*, Thomas Bleck, MD, FCCM[a,b,c,d]

KEYWORDS

- Neurocritical care • Critical care • Neurology • Head trauma • Intracranial pressure

KEY POINTS

- Head trauma is a major aspect of neurocritical care, and the management of cranial injuries can be traced back to 2000 BC.
- The first contemporary neurointensive care units using mechanical ventilation developed after the poliomyelitis epidemic of the 1920s.
- Modern neurointensive care units use multiple modalities to monitor a diverse patient population.
- The Neurocritical Care Society was founded in 2002 and is a multidisciplinary organization dedicated to progress in the field of neurocritical care and improvement in patient outcomes.

HISTORICAL ASPECTS

The history of neurocritical care begins in antiquity, as documented in the Edwin Smith surgical papyrus. This text, named for a nineteenth century Egyptologist who purchased the document in Luxor or Thebes in 1862, is an unfinished textbook on bodily injuries written *circa* 1700 BC. It is believed to be a copy of an original article written 1000 years prior and describes 48 case reports, including 27 head injuries and 6 spinal cord injuries, many with documented interventions by the investigator. The Edwin Smith papyrus is remarkable in that it not only gives the first anatomic description of the brain, cerebrospinal fluid, and meninges but also describes conditions such as tetanus and aphasia.[1,2]

Although this extraordinary work gives us a view of ancient medical practices, it does not mention the earliest known neurosurgical procedure of trepanation, which

Disclosures: None.
[a] Department of Neurological Sciences, Rush University Medical Center, 600 South Paulina Street, Chicago, IL 60612, USA; [b] Department of Neurosurgery, Rush University Medical Center, 600 South Paulina Street, Chicago, IL 60612, USA; [c] Department of Anesthesiology, Rush University Medical Center, 600 South Paulina Street, Chicago, IL 60612, USA; [d] Department of Internal Medicine, Rush University Medical Center, 600 South Paulina Street, Chicago, IL 60612, USA
* Corresponding author.
E-mail address: georgiakorbakis@gmail.com

Crit Care Clin 30 (2014) 657–671
http://dx.doi.org/10.1016/j.ccc.2014.06.001   criticalcare.theclinics.com
0749-0704/14/$ – see front matter © 2014 Elsevier Inc. All rights reserved.

appears to have originated in the Neolithic Era after the discovery of a trephined skull dating back to 10,000 BC. Hippocrates, frequently hailed as the "father of medicine," clearly documented and advocated trepanation as a management for certain head injuries including skull fractures and contusions. He also documented neuroanatomic observations, categorized different skull fractures, suggested treatment for such injuries, and recognized deleterious complications such as fever and inflammation.[3] About 300 years later, Aulus Aurelius Cornelius Celsus of Alexandria promoted the work of Hippocrates, but additionally described epidural and subdural hematoma evacuation via trepanation. In the 2nd century AD, another titan in the field of medicine, Galen of Pergamon, further expanded on the technique of trepanation and described innovative new tools.[4] This ancient era also heralded the initial management for spinal cord injury, and Hippocrates is credited for one of these early treatments: traction. By using an extension bench he was able to reduce spinal deformities. Celsus and Galen further advanced the understanding of the pathophysiology of spinal cord injury by recognizing that damage to the "spinal marrow" or cord, and not the vertebrae, leads to deficits.[5]

The medieval times following the flourishing of science and medicine in the Greco-Roman epoch lacked major advances, excepting those described by one famous Persian intellectual, Avicenna. His *Canon of Medicine* was used as a medical text throughout Europe up until the eighteenth century,[6] and he may have been the first to realize that stroke was due to blockage of the cerebral vessels, offering remedies for management of acute stroke including venesection.[7]

MECHANICAL VENTILATION AND THE BIRTH OF CRITICAL CARE MEDICINE

A complete discussion of the history of mechanical ventilation is beyond the scope of this article; however, many key elements to the development of artificial respiration are relevant to critical care medicine as a subspecialty, and particularly neurocritical care. Galen first described using a bellows to ventilate a dead animal artificially through the trachea; later, the Renaissance physician Andreas Vesalius documented the use of a tracheostomy with artificial respiration by inserting a reed tube into the trachea of animals and blowing in air to observe the heart and thoracic cavity during vivisection.[8] Over a century later, in 1744, the first report of positive pressure ventilation by mouth-to-mouth resuscitation was described by the surgeon William Tossach during the successful revival of a suffocated miner.[9] Around the same time, several methods regarding the resuscitation of humans were in practice, including insufflating tobacco smoke through the anus and rolling a barrel against a victim's thorax.[10,11]

The next great stride was in respiratory physiology with the discovery of carbon dioxide by Joseph Black. He demonstrated that carbon dioxide was the product of respiration through experiments with caustic alkali.[12] The discovery of oxygen by Joseph Priestley and Carl Wilhelm Scheele soon followed through tests involving heating mercuric oxide.[13] Antoine-Laurent de Lavoisier repeated these experiments and named the gas "oxygen." He also realized that oxygen was necessary for respiration or "internal combustion."[14] By the end of the eighteenth century, bellows and pistons were favored over mouth-to-mouth resuscitation for both aesthetic reasons and concern over lack of effectiveness when using expired air containing carbon dioxide.[11] Despite this trend, positive pressure ventilation was strongly criticized after experiments on drowned animals in the 1800s demonstrated emphysema when the lungs were inflated forcibly, and thus this practice fell out of favor.[9,15]

In the early nineteenth century, attention was directed toward negative pressure ventilation. Dr Dalziel introduced the tank respirator, which enclosed the patient in a cylindrical tube and used bellows to reduce the pressure within the tank to subatmospheric levels.[15] In 1929, Drinker and Shaw published their work on a new tank respirator that used electrically operated pumps to create negative and positive pressure within the tank.[16] This respirator became known as the "iron lung" and was used extensively throughout the United States to provide ventilatory support for respiratory paralysis during the poliomyelitis epidemic of the late 1940s.[17] The poliomyelitis epidemic in Copenhagen in 1952 prompted the use of intermittent positive pressure ventilation. Copenhagen was overwhelmed by a large number of bulbar cases of poliomyelitis with a mortality rate of 80%.[18,19] Primary credit is given to anesthesiologist, Bjørn Ibsen, who treated a patient with tracheotomy followed by manual positive pressure bag ventilation using humidified oxygen. This technique was applied to several patients, and a large staff, including 250 medical students, worked in relays to provide uninterrupted ventilation for patients. The mortality rate in Copenhagen was cut to 39%.[18] Knowledge spread throughout Europe, and quickly intermittent positive pressure ventilation became standard practice.[17,20]

The Copenhagen poliomyelitis epidemic provided the catalyst for the development of dedicated respiratory care units—the first true intensive care units (ICUs)—to treat patients with respiratory failure of various causes, although Florence Nightingale is customarily regarded as the first to have established an ICU during the Crimean War. Nightingale clustered the sicker patients in a "monitoring unit." Dr Dandy Walker created a specialized unit for his post-operative neurosurgical patients at the Johns Hopkins Hospital in 1929.[21]

With the subsequent development of respiratory and cardiac ICUs, a decrease in mortality rate between mechanically ventilated patients treated in traditional general hospitals compared with those in new ICUs was quickly identified and provided convincing evidence for the establishment of these units, despite higher costs.[22] In 1971, the Society of Critical Care Medicine was founded to promote the field and define core competencies. The 3 founding physicians came from different medical specialties: cardiology, anesthesiology, and trauma surgery.[21] ICUs today remain diverse, and neurocritical care units represent yet another important subspecialty linking the care of the damaged nervous system to other organs.

HEAD TRAUMA

Traumatic brain injury (TBI) has gained much attention in the news recently, especially regarding sports-related injuries; however, severe TBI due to injuries sustained during periods of war has been a topic of study since antiquity. One of the main indications for trepanation is thought to have been TBI. Trepanation could be performed by scraping, grooving, or boring and cutting, as was performed by the Greeks, using an instrument called a trypanon. Interestingly, many of the ancient skulls discovered showed postoperative changes in the bone, indicating survival after the procedure. Hippocrates was the first to systematically document skull fractures and emphasized the importance of history taking and careful physical examination.[23] Rhazes, a Muslim physician practicing in the ninth century, was the first to define concussion in the modern sense by recognizing that brain injury could occur without skull fracture. In the fourteenth century, Guy de Chauliac further elaborated this concept. He described the term commotio cerebri, a transient cerebral dysfunction caused by the brain being shaken and not necessarily related to structural pathology.[24] The next great work regarding head trauma, *Tractatus de Fractura Calvae sive Cranei* (*Treatise on Fractures of the Calvaria or Cranium*) was written by Berengario da Carpi in the sixteenth century. He noted the difference between injuries involving the dura mater, as opposed to the pia mater (the latter also involved the underlying brain parenchyma), and described surgical treatments for head trauma including a description of contemporary instruments.[25]

The prevalence of wars in the next few centuries along with the increased use of firearms during warfare ushered in a new era of TBI medicine. The American Civil War (1861–1865) saw a great deal of head injury but unfortunately, due to lack of aseptic technique, surgery frequently met with significant infection and subsequent mortality. The medical "pocket manuals" of the time served as guides for military doctors. They classified injuries into blunt or penetrating wounds and distinguished between immediate concussion and delayed compression, now recognized as herniation. Advances in anesthesia, such as the use of ether, allowed advances in surgery as well.[26] World War I (1914–1918) advanced the treatment of brain wounds as both the Allied and Central powers dealt with trench warfare and focal brain injury due to smaller ammunition. The English neurosurgeon Percy Sargent and neurologist Gordon Holmes emphasized the importance of a detailed neurologic examination before operation, gave indications for different procedures, and described increases in intracranial pressure (ICP) as well as the underlying causes and treatment.[27] The topic of increased ICP was further expanded on by Harvey Cushing, who went to France in 1917 as part of the war effort. Dr Cushing's experiences in Europe rapidly advanced the field of neurosurgery and the surgical treatment of TBI by addressing hemostasis and aseptic technique. Additionally, his contributions regarding the use of radiographs and the Riva-Rocci pneumatic device for recording blood pressure during anesthesia were particularly valuable.[28] George Tabuteau was a proponent of the then-controversial issue of opening the dura to remove clot, which subsequently lowered infection rates and improved outcomes.[29] Robert Bárány, a surgeon in the Austro-Hungarian army, described the importance of primary wound closure after thorough debridement to prevent infection.[30] Over the remainder of the twentieth century, advances in evacuation times from the battlefield and improvement in our understanding of the pathophysiology and monitoring of TBI have decreased the mortality rates of head wounds from 74% in the Crimean War to 10% in the Korean and Vietnam wars.[23]

TBI in the civilian population remains a serious epidemiologic issue with an annual incidence of 1.7 million and a mortality rate of 52,000 per year.[31] In 1996, the Brain Trauma Foundation published the first set of guidelines for the management of severe TBI. These were most recently revised in 2007. Current recommendations focus on avoiding hypotension and hypoxia while managing ICP and maintaining cerebral perfusion and oxygenation.[32] Adherence to these guidelines significantly improves survival among TBI patients.[33,34]

INTRACRANIAL PRESSURE

Assessment and management of ICP remains one of the main responsibilities for neurointensivists practicing today. In 1901, Cushing published a landmark study demonstrating the "Cushing response:" a triad of hypertension, bradycardia, and irregular respirations related to intracranial hypertension. Increasing ICP in dogs via infusion of a salt solution directly into the subdural space and recording several physiologic measures, Cushing noted a direct correlation of the increase in arterial blood pressure with ICP elevation and determined this was a regulatory mechanism to maintain perfusion to the brainstem. The recognition of this triad of symptoms remains crucial to clinical intensive care.[35]

Evaluation of elevated ICP was traditionally assessed by clinical examination, measurement of vital signs, and inference from lumbar puncture. In 1953, Ryder and colleagues[36] published a case series recording cerebrospinal fluid pressure continuously in a few patients following acute brain injury, and in 1965 Lundberg and colleagues[37] published the first report of continuous ICP monitoring using ventricular cannula in patients with TBI and nontraumatic cases of intracranial hypertension.[38] This article demonstrated the variations in ICP following head injury and provided a targeted approach for the management of elevated ICP. Continuous ICP monitoring remains an integral aspect in the care of the critically ill neurologic patient, extending beyond traumatic injuries and is discussed in a later section.

Although identification of elevated ICP is critical, treatment options are scarce and reveal the tremendous gaps in our current knowledge of the pathophysiology and management of intracranial hypertension. Cushing was truly a pioneer in this field and was the first to describe palliative subtemporal decompression to relieve elevated ICP before brain tumor resection, thus lowering the risk of herniation during the resection.[39] Decompressive hemicraniectomy remains one of the few tools to definitively manage elevated ICP. A modern application of this concept frequently encountered in neurologic ICUs today is evident in the recent publications of 3 randomized controlled trials from Europe (HAMLET, DESTINY, and DECIMAL) showing that early decompressive hemicraniectomy reduces mortality in patients with large hemispheric ischemic stroke.[40]

The use of chemical agents to lower elevated ICP was developed in the early twentieth century. In 1919, Weed and McKibben[41] published a study on ICP changes following intravenous injection of solutions with varying concentrations. They recorded cerebrospinal fluid (CSF) pressures in cats and demonstrated a sustained elevation following infusion of hypotonic distilled water and conversely, a marked and rapid decrease in ICP with administration of hypertonic saline and other highly concentrated salt solutions. Fremont-Smith and Forbes[42] found intravenous hypertonic urea lowered ICP in animals. Initially used in humans in the 1950s, urea soon fell out of favor due to difficulties in preparation.[43] Mannitol was first studied in dogs in 1961; subsequently, Wise and Chater[44] published their report of lowering CSF pressure in 24 patients with various causes of intracranial hypertension using mannitol. In the 1990s, there was a resurgence of interest in other hypertonic solutions after several studies demonstrated improved survival in patients treated with hypertonic saline mixed with dextran for hemorrhagic shock following trauma, termed "small volume resuscitation." Some investigators deemed the improvement to be due to rapid increase in systemic arterial pressure and reduction in cerebral edema, with subsequent increase in cerebral perfusion.[45,46] The use of hyperosmolar agents either as continuous infusions or as boluses is still in practice today in the management of elevated ICP.

Since the 1930s, the correlation between barbiturates and lowered ICP has been identified, by their effect on reducing cerebral metabolism.[47] Their use, however, was limited due to side effects of hypovolemia and respiratory depression. In 1988, Eisenberg and colleagues[48] compared patients with elevated ICP receiving conventional therapy (hyperventilation, neuromuscular junction blockade, sedation, mannitol, and ventricular drainage) to those receiving conventional therapy plus pentobarbital and found high-dose pentobarbital to be an effective adjunctive therapy for elevated ICP. Currently, high-dose barbiturates used to achieve a burst-suppression pattern on continuous electroencephalography (EEG) are used to lower ICP in medically refractory cases.

Therapeutic hypothermia has also been used for the management of elevated ICP. The most evidence comes from TBI studies where it is used in medically refractory cases.[49] It has also been effective at controlling ICP in acute hepatic failure.[50]

NEUROMONITORING

The field of neurocritical care is relatively young but has quickly evolved over the last 30 years to involve a multidisciplinary approach to the management of acute neurologic injury. The term "multimodal monitoring" refers to measuring and recording neurospecific variables in real time, in addition to the patient's cardiac and pulmonary status.

The oldest and most dependable of these variables is the neurologic examination. Vigilant bedside monitoring for neurologic deterioration is difficult but remains vital in the care of the neurologically ill patient. Serial clinical neurologic examinations remain crucial in the ICU. Although several coma scales have been documented,[51] the Glasgow coma scale is one of the most commonly used tools in the neuroICU. Introduced in 1974 by Teasdale and Jeannett, it is extensively used worldwide to classify the level of consciousness. Clinical parameters measure the best motor, verbal, and eye opening responses; a summed score of 8 or less suggests coma and the need for intubation.[52] This scale has become increasingly useful in communication during patient transfer (eg, from a community hospital to a tertiary care center).[53]

More recently, the FOUR (Full Outline UnResponsiveness) score was developed by Wijdicks and colleagues,[54] assigning a score from 1 to 4 to each of 4 components: eye response, motor response, brainstem reflexes, and respiration. This score was validated in 2005 and allows for greater neurologic detail during evaluation, remaining testable in intubated patients as well.

Monitoring and measuring changes in ICP are crucial parts of neurocritical care and are fundamental in the management of patients with subarachnoid hemorrhage (SAH), TBI, hydrocephalus, stroke, central nervous system infection, and hepatic failure. The importance of ICP was recognized over 2 centuries ago by Alexander Monro, and advances in monitoring and managing ICP and related measures are in continuous evolution.[55] Claude-Nicolas Le Cat first documented the placement of an external ventricular drain after specially devising a cannula with a stopple that was placed in the lateral ventricle and used to drain small volumes of CSF in an infant with hydrocephalus.[56] William Williams Keen, Emil Theodor Kocher, and Hermann Tillmanns made significant advances in approach and aseptic technique.[57] Throughout the twentieth century, advances in materials proved most noteworthy from horsehairs and catgut to metals and modern plastic catheters. However, as mentioned previously, Lundberg was one of the first physicians to continuously measure and document ICP using a ventricular catheter—this procedure continues to be used in neuroICUs today.[37] This device is easily placed at the bedside using anatomic landmarks and has the added benefit of being able to treat elevations in ICP via drainage of CSF. The most significant complications include malposition, occlusion, hemorrhage, and infection. Current studies examine the use of silver or antibiotic-coated catheters to reduce the risk of ventriculitis, but a consensus has yet to be determined.[58,59]

Fiberoptic, transducer-tipped monitors were developed in the 1980s and experience with these devices continues to build. Again, the device is easily inserted at the bedside and can be left in place for continuous ICP measurement. The intraparenchymal monitors have lower complication rates, but major issues include transducer disconnection and drift.[60] Additionally, a significant fraction of patients with an intraparenchymal monitor still require external ventricular drainage placement to treat elevated ICP.[61]

Several other modalities have been developed to continuously monitor the neurologically ill patient. EEG, traditionally thought of for the analysis of seizures, provides a continuous, noninvasive approach to determine brain function, specifically cerebral ischemia. In the 1970s, changes in cerebral blood flow during carotid endarterectomy were noted to correlate with EEG changes, specifically a replacement of faster alpha range frequencies for slower theta and delta range components.[62] Quantitative EEG transforms EEG waves into numerical values that are compressed over a large period of time to form visual graphs, allowing the reader to compare one cerebral hemisphere to the other. This technique has been increasingly used in the management of SAH to detect delayed cerebral ischemia in the comatose patient and has shown accuracy in predicting ischemia before clinical or radiographic changes.[63,64] It provides the added benefit of continuous monitoring, rather than the routine daily transcranial Doppler ultrasounds, which only provide data for one time point. Quantitative EEG continues to be limited by artifact and requires an experienced electroencephalographer to interpret. Use of intracortical EEG via a depth electrode has recently been documented in 5 poor-grade SAH patients and shows some promise in detecting ischemia by reducing EEG artifact.[65]

There are several new methods for measuring cerebral oxygenation and a few will be discussed here. Near infrared spectroscopy was described in the 1970s and was clinically used to monitor cerebral ischemia during carotid and cardiac surgery. The device measures the transmission and absorption of near infrared frequency light and is used as an indirect measure of oxygenation. The monitor is noninvasive and, although it has been used with increasing frequency in SAH and TBI patients, the research is limited[66] and sometimes contradictory.[67]

Jugular venous bulb oximetry has been used to measure jugular venous oxygen saturation, which is the result of oxygen delivery to the brain minus the cerebral metabolic rate of oxygen. It has mainly been applied to comatose patients following TBI to identify global cerebral ischemia, and desaturations have been associated with poor neurologic outcome.[68] There are several risks with the use of jugular venous bulb oximetry, including insertion complications and low sensitivity.[69]

Brain tissue oxygen monitors were first used in the 1990s and involve insertion of a small catheter directly into the brain parenchyma. Benefits of these monitors include that they can be placed in an area of interest to determine regional ischemia. They have been mainly studied in TBI, SAH, and large hemispheric infarctions and offer real-time information that can guide management of these patients.[70]

Since 1992, cerebral microdialysis, a technique for continuous monitoring of cerebral chemistry and metabolism, has been used in neurologic ICUs. A thin catheter with a semipermeable membrane is inserted into the brain parenchyma and perfusate is infused. Chemicals from the interstitial space diffuse through the membrane, and the fluid is collected and analyzed. The main markers investigated are glucose, lactate, pyruvate, and glutamate.[71] Levels and ratios of these metabolic substances have been studied and correlation with outcomes after severe TBI has been made. Additionally, changes in these values have been shown to be early predictors of vasospasm in SAH.[72] Microdialysis has furthered our understanding of brain energy metabolism following severe neurologic injury and may be used as a tool in the future for the direct delivery of substances to damaged tissue or for measuring drug concentrations in brain tissue.[73]

BRAIN DEATH

With the increasing use of mechanical ventilation in the 1950s, patients who would have previously died from respiratory arrest were being kept alive in ICUs around the world; this resulted in a widely cited French study on *coma dépassé* (a state beyond coma or irreversible coma) by Mollaret and Goulet published in 1959.[74] This study documented 23 patients who lost consciousness and other brainstem function and reflexes but maintained a heartbeat while being kept on mechanical ventilation. This study later prompted an *ad hoc* committee of anesthesiologists, neurologists, neurosurgeons, ethicists, public health and biochemistry professors, as well as transplant surgeons to convene at Harvard Medical School and define criteria for what was then termed brain death.[75] The clinical criteria included unresponsivity, absence of movement and brainstem reflexes, areflexia, and apnea in the context of an identified cause for coma.[76] In 1976, the Conference of Medical Royal Colleges and their Faculties in the United Kingdom issued a statement defining brain death as the loss of all brainstem reflexes.[77] Shortly thereafter, the President's Commission for the Study of Ethical Problems in Medicine and Biomedical and Behavioral Research published the Uniform Determination of Death Act providing either cardiopulmonary or neurologic criteria for the legal determination of death.[78]

The American Academy of Neurology conducted an evidence-based review and published guidelines defining death by neurologic criteria in 1995 focusing on the clinical examination and apnea testing.[79] Although all 50 states have adopted the Uniform Determination of Death Act, there remains great variability among different states and different institutions regarding the guidelines for diagnosing brain death;[80] this holds true regarding the diagnostic criteria for brain death worldwide as well.[81] Ancillary testing such as cerebral angiography, EEG, transcranial Doppler sonography, and nuclear imaging are available, but there are no clear guidelines regarding their use.

This concept of brain death remains controversial. Some have argued that the Harvard report was devised as a way to ensure organ donors in the new era of transplant medicine. Others have taken a more philosophic approach and have promoted the term "total brain failure" instead.[82]

CARDIOPULMONARY RESUSCITATION AND HYPOTHERMIA FOR CARDIAC ARREST

A synopsis regarding the evolution of critical care medicine as a specialty would not be complete without a discussion of cardiopulmonary resuscitation (CPR); however, details regarding positive pressure ventilation were discussed earlier. Peter Safar, an anesthesiologist named the "father of CPR," first introduced the concept of mouth-to-mouth resuscitation with the head-tilt-chin-lift method to open the patient's airway, publishing his work in a landmark study in JAMA in 1958.[83] Combining the findings of closed-chest cardiac massage by W B Kouwenhoven, James Jude, and G Guy Knickerbocker, which showed that a pulse could be generated on dogs by external chest compressions,[84] Safar united this information and came up with the "ABCs" of basic life support. Safar realized that patients surviving cardiac arrest and his own post-operative patients needed closer monitoring and thus established the first multidisciplinary physician-staffed ICU in the United States at Baltimore City Hospital in 1958.[85] Dr Safar's attention then turned toward cerebral resuscitation following cardiopulmonary arrest and included investigations into hypothermia.[17]

Hypothermia had been used in the 1940s to reduce cerebral edema during neurosurgery, and it was around that time that interest began to build regarding the use of hypothermia following cardiac arrest, with case series publishing successful outcomes in patients who were cooled.[86] In February 2002, two studies published in the New England Journal of Medicine demonstrated improved neurologic outcomes in patients treated with hypothermia shortly after cardiac arrest.[87,88] The 2010 practice guidelines for Advanced Cardiac Life Support include induced hypothermia to a temperature of 32°C to 34°C for a period of 12 or 24 hours in the algorithm for post–cardiac arrest care in a patient who does not follow commands following return of spontaneous circulation.[89] In many institutions, the neurocritical care team is responsible for therapeutic hypothermia following cardiac arrest.

FUTURE DIRECTION

Since its inception, the field of neurocritical care has grown dramatically. Much of this article has focused on TBI and multimodal monitoring where the goal is to prevent secondary injury. An emerging specialty, neurocritical care bioinformatics, attempts to use all the data gathered through multimodal monitoring and analyze these parameters at the bedside in real time to aid in decision-making for complicated cases;[90] this may prove to be an exciting new development as we continue to understand the complex physiologic relationships following brain injury.

Although over the last several years we have learned that oxygen free radicals are a common pathway leading to neuronal dysfunction, further research is needed to identify targets to prevent cerebral reperfusion injury. One such target includes modulation of the mitochondrial permeability transition pore.[91] More practical studies are currently underway as well. For example, the ATACH II study is designed to determine the ideal systolic blood pressure goal for patients suffering acute intracranial hemorrhage.[92]

Several advances have been made in ischemic stroke in the last few decades. The major advance to date was in 1995 with the publication of the National Institute of Neurologic Disorders and Stroke rt-PA trial supporting the use of intravenous tissue plasminogen activator (t-PA) for ischemic strokes, which demonstrated improved clinical outcomes in treated patients at 3 months.[93] A major role of the neurocritical care unit now is to admit patients who have received rt-PA for close monitoring for at least 24 hours given the risk of bleeding. With the invention of several clot retrieval devices, endovascular treatment of stroke in addition to t-PA was becoming popular; recently, however, 3 studies (MR RESCUE, IMS III, SYNTHESIS Expansion) have not shown any benefit in clinical outcomes for ischemic stroke patients undergoing endovascular treatment with or without rt-PA. Nevertheless, further studies are in process to identify stroke patients who may benefit from endovascular therapies.[94]

Patients in the neuroICU also have nonvascular pathologies, particularly the immune-mediated disorders. Guillain-Barré syndrome or acute inflammatory demyelinating polyneuropathy is perhaps one of the more common immune-mediated disorders requiring ICU admission when neuromuscular respiratory failure or autonomic instability occurs. Intravenous immunoglobulin or plasmapheresis is the preferred treatment.[95] An interesting variant, the Miller-Fisher syndrome, was described in the 1950s as a triad of ophthalmoplegia, ataxia, and areflexia.[96] Around the same time, Bickerstaff proposed a brainstem encephalitis with patients suffering from ophthalmoplegia, ataxia, and impaired consciousness.[97] Both diseases tended to occur after an infection and later the antiganglioside antibody GQ1b was discovered in both Miller-Fisher syndrome and Bickerstaff's encephalitis. The 2 syndromes are now felt to represent a spectrum of the same disease process.[98]

Another great stride in antibody-mediated diseases is seen with the paraneoplastic syndromes. Onconeural antibodies were first discovered in the 1980s and some classic examples include Lambert-Eaton myasthenic syndrome, subacute cerebellar degeneration, and dermatomyositis. These syndromes are believed to be caused by an immune response directed against neuronal proteins expressed by a malignant tumor.[99] Recently, an anti-N-methyl-D-aspartate receptor antibody was discovered in young women presenting with prominent psychiatric symptoms, seizures, orofacial dyskinesias, dysautonomia, and decreased level of consciousness, who were later found to have ovarian teratomas. Although this condition can be lethal, several patients who required ventilatory support, immunotherapy, and tumor resection survived with marked neurologic improvement.[100] Several antibodies against neuronal antigens continue to be discovered, and prompt identification and tumor screening are crucial.

SUMMARY

Neurocritical care is a diverse and fascinating field that has quickly blossomed from a small group of interested physicians in the 1980s to an established subspecialty encompassing doctors trained in neurology, neurosurgery, internal medicine, and emergency medicine. In 2002 the Neurocritical Care Society was founded in San Francisco, CA by a small group of neurointensivists. The group held its inaugural meeting in Phoenix, AZ in 2003. The United Council of Neurologic Subspecialties, founded in 2005, formally recognized neurocritical care as a subspecialty fellowship.[101] As diagnostic and therapeutic modalities continue to be developed, it is recognized that highly trained individuals with a profound understanding of cerebral physiology and metabolism are crucial. NeuroICUs are now present in most major medical centers across the United States, and several studies have demonstrated improved outcomes when neurologically ill patients are cared for by specially trained staff.[102,103] As the field continues to grow, and with the support of an established professional society, advances will hopefully continue along with development of new technologies and improved clinical trial design. However, the roots of neurocritical care—mainly improving outcomes in disorders of the nervous system—can be traced back for thousands of years.

REFERENCES

1. Hughes JT. The Edwin Smith surgical papyrus: an analysis of the first case reports of spinal cord injuries. Paraplegia 1988;26:71–82.
2. Breasted JH. The Edwin Smith surgical papyrus, published in facsimile and hieroglyphic transliteration with translation and commentary. Chicago: The University of Chicago Press; 1930.
3. Kelly EC. Hippocrates on injuries of the head. In: Krieger RE, editor. Classics of neurology. Huntington (NY): R.E. Krieger Pub Co; 1949.
4. Kshettry VR, Mindea SA, Batjer HH. The management of cranial injuries in antiquity and beyond. Neurosurg Focus 2007;23(1):E8.
5. Lifshutz J, Colohan A. A brief history of therapy for traumatic spinal cord injury. Neurosurg Focus 2004;16(1):E5.
6. Rahimi SY, McDonnell DE, Ahmadian A, et al. Medieval neurosurgery: contributions from the Middle East, Spain, and Persia. Neurosurg Focus 2007;23(1):E14.
7. Zargaran A, Zarshenas MM, Karimi A, et al. Management of stroke as described by Ibn Sina (Avicenna) in the Canon of Medicine. Int J Cardiol 2013;169(4):233–7.
8. Vallejo-Manzur F, Perkins Y, Varon J, et al. The resuscitation greats: Andreas Vesalius, the concept of an artificial airway. Resuscitation 2003;56:3–7.
9. Baker AB. Artificial respiration, the history of an idea. Med Hist 1971;15:336–51.
10. Lee RV. Cardiopulmonary resuscitation in the eighteenth century: a historical perspective on present practice. J Hist Med Allied Sci 1972;27(4):418–33.
11. Trubuhovich RV. History of mouth-to-mouth rescue breathing, Part 2: the 18th century. Crit Care Resusc 2006;8(2):157–71.
12. Foregger R. Joseph Black and the identification of carbon dioxide. Anesthesiology 1957;18(2):257–64.

13. West JB. Joseph Priestley, oxygen, and the Enlightenment. Am J Physiol Lung Cell Mol Physiol 2014;306(2):L111–9.
14. Underwood EA. Lavoisier and the history of respiration. Proc R Soc Med 1944; 37(6):247–62.
15. Price JL. The evolution of breathing machines. Med Hist 1962;6(1):67–72.
16. Drinker P, Shaw LA. An apparatus for the prolonged administration of artificial respiration. J Clin Invest 1929;7:229–47.
17. Rosengart MR. Critical care medicine: landmarks and legends. Surg Clin North Am 2006;86:1305–21.
18. Lassen H. The epidemic of poliomyelitis in Copenhagen, 1952. Proc R Soc Med 1954;47(1):67–71.
19. Lassen H. A preliminary report on the 1952 epidemic of poliomyelitis in Copenhagen with special reference to the treatment of acute respiratory insufficiency. Lancet 1953;1(6749):37–41.
20. Engström CG. Treatment of severe cases of respiratory paralysis by the Engström universal respirator. Br Med J 1954;2(4889):666–9.
21. Grenvik A, Pinsky MR. Evolution of the intensive care unit as a clinical center and critical care medicine as a discipline. Crit Care Clin 2009;25:239–50.
22. Rogers RM, Weiler C, Ruppenthal B. Impact of the respiratory intensive care unit of survival of patients with acute respiratory failure. Chest 1972;62(1):94–7.
23. Rose FC. The history of head injuries: an overview. J Hist Neurosci 1997;6(2): 154–80.
24. McCrory PF, Berkovic SF. Concussion: the history of clinical and pathophysiological concepts and misconceptions. Neurology 2001;57:2283–9.
25. Di Ieva A, Gaetani P, Matula C, et al. Berengario da Capri: a pioneer in neurotraumatology. J Neurosurg 2011;114(5):1461–70.
26. Kaufman HH. Treatment of head injuries in the American Civil War. J Neurosurg 1993;78:838–45.
27. Sargent P, Holmes G. Preliminary notes on the treatment of the cranial injuries of warfare. Br Med J 1915;1(2830):537–41.
28. Kinsman M, Pendleton C, Quinones-Hinojosa A, et al. Harvey Cushing's early experience with the surgical treatment of head trauma. J Hist Neurosci 2013;22:96–115.
29. Tabuteau GG. The treatment of gunshot wounds of the head, based on a series of ninety-five cases. Br Med J 1915;2(2857):501–2.
30. Carey ME. Cushing and the treatment of brain wounds during World War I. J Neurosurg 2011;114:1495–501.
31. Faul M, Xu L, Wald MM, et al. Traumatic brain injury in the United States: emergency department visits, hospitalizations and deaths 2002–2006. Atlanta (GA): Centers for Disease Control and Prevention, National Center for Injury Prevention and Control; 2010.
32. Brain Trauma Foundation, American Association of Neurological Surgeons, Congress of Neurological Surgeons. Guidelines for the management of severe traumatic brain injury. J Neurotrauma 2007;24:S1–106.
33. Talving P, Karamanos E, Teixeira PG, et al. Intracranial pressure monitoring in severe head injury: compliance with Brain Trauma Foundation guidelines and effect on outcomes: a prospective study. J Neurosurg 2013;119(5):1248–54.
34. Gerber LM, Chiu YL, Carney N, et al. Marked reduction in mortality in patients with severe traumatic brain injury. J Neurosurg 2013;119:1583–90.
35. Cushing H. Concerning a definite regulatory mechanism of the vasomotor centre which controls blood pressure during cerebral compression. Johns Hopkins Hospital Bulletin 1901;12:290–2.

36. Ryder H, Espey F, Kimbell F, et al. The mechanism of change in cerebrospinal fluid pressure following an induced change in the volume of the fluid space. J Lab Clin Med 1953;41:428–35.

37. Lundberg N, Troupp H, Lorin H. Continuous recording of the ventricular-fluid pressure in patients with severe acute traumatic brain injury: a preliminary report. J Neurosurg 1965;22:581–90.

38. Lundberg N. Continuous recording and control of ventricular fluid pressure in neurosurgical practice. Acta Psychiatr Scand Suppl 1960;36(149):1–193.

39. Greenblatt SH. The crucial decade: modern neurosurgery's definitive development in Harvey Cushing's early research and practice, 1900 to 1910. J Neurosurg 1997;87:964–71.

40. Vahedi K, Hofmeijer J, Juettler E, et al. Early decompressive surgery in malignant infarction of the middle cerebral artery: a pooled analysis of three randomized controlled trials. Lancet Neurol 2007;6:215–22.

41. Weed LH, McKibben PS. Pressure changes in the cerebro-spinal fluid following intravenous injection of solutions of various concentrations. Am J Physiol 1919; 48(40):512–30.

42. Fremont-Smith F, Forbes HS. Intra-ocular and intracranial pressure: an experimental study. Arch Neurol Psychiatry 1927;18:550–64.

43. Javid M, Settlage P. Effect of urea on cerebrospinal fluid pressure in human subjects: preliminary report. J Am Med Assoc 1956;160:943–9.

44. Wise BL, Chater N. The value of hypertonic mannitol solution in decreasing brain mass and lowering cerebrospinal-fluid pressure. J Neurosurg 1962;19(12):1038–43.

45. Wade CE, Grady JJ, Kramer GC, et al. Individual patient cohort analysis of the efficacy of hypertonic saline/dextran in patients with traumatic brain injury and hypotension. J Trauma 1997;42(5 Suppl):S61–5.

46. Qureshi AI, Suarez JI. Use of hypertonic saline solutions in treatment of cerebral edema and intracranial hypertension. Crit Care Med 2000;28(9):3301–13.

47. Horsley JS. The intracranial pressure during barbital narcosis. Lancet 1937; 229(5916):141–3.

48. Eisenberg HM, Frankowski RF, Contant CF, et al. High-dose barbiturate control of elevated intracranial pressure in patients with severe head injury. J Neurosurg 1988;69:15–23.

49. Sadaka F, Veremakis C. Therapeutic hypothermia for the management of intracranial hypertension in severe traumatic brain injury: a systematic review. Brain Inj 2012;26:899–908.

50. Jalan R, Damink SW, Deutz NE, et al. Moderate hypothermia for uncontrolled intracranial hypertension in acute liver failure. Lancet 1999;354:1164–8.

51. Bordini AL, Luiz TF, Fernandes M, et al. Coma scales: a historical review. Arq Neuropsiquiatr 2010;68(6):930–7.

52. Teasdale G, Jennett B. Assessment of coma and impaired consciousness: a practical scale. Lancet 1974;2:81–4.

53. Wijdicks EF. The clinical practice of critical care neurology. Philadelphia: Lippincott-Raven; 1997.

54. Wijdicks EF, Bamlet WR, Maramattom BV, et al. Validation of a new coma scale: the FOUR score. Ann Neurol 2005;58:585–93.

55. Wang VY, Manley GT. Intracranial pressure monitoring. In: Winn HR, editor. Youmans neurological surgery. Philadephia: Elsevier; 2011. p. 424–8.

56. Le Cat CN. A new trocar for the puncture in the hydrocephalus, and for other evacuations, which are necessary to be made at different times. Philos Trans R Soc Lond 1751;157:267–72.

57. Srinivasan VM, O'Neill BR, Jho D, et al. The history of external ventricular drainage. J Neurosurg 2014;120:228–36.
58. Keong NC, Bulters DO, Richards HK, et al. The SILVER (Silver Impregnated Line versus EVD Randomized Trial): a double-blind, prospective, randomized, controlled trial of an intervention to reduce the rate of external ventricular drain infection. Neurosurgery 2012;71:394–404.
59. Wang X, Dong Y, Qi XQ, et al. Clinical review: efficacy of antimicrobial-impregnated catheters in external ventricular drainage - a systematic review and meta-analysis. Crit Care 2013;17:234.
60. Kasotakis G, Michailidou M, Bramos A, et al. Intraparenchymal vs extracranial ventricular drain intracranial pressure monitors in traumatic brain injury: less is more? J Am Coll Surg 2012;214:950–7.
61. Bekar A, Doğan S, Abaş F, et al. Risk factors and complications of intracranial pressure monitoring with a fiberoptic device. J Clin Neurosci 2009;16(2):236–40.
62. Sharbrough FW, Messick JM, Sundt TM. Correlation of continuous electroencephalograms with cerebral blood flow measurements during carotid endarterectomy. Stroke 1973;4:674–83.
63. Foreman B, Claassen J. Quantitative EEG for the detection of brain ischemia. Critical Care 2012;16(20):216.
64. Rosenthal ES. The utility of EEG, SSEP and other neurophysiologic tools to guide neurocritical care. Neurotherapeutics 2012;9:24–36.
65. Stuart RM, Waziri A, Weintraub D, et al. Intracortical EEG for the detection of vasospasm in patients with poor-grade subarachnoid hemorrhage. Neurocrit Care 2010;13:355–8.
66. Ghosh A, Elwell C, Smith M. Cerebral near-infrared spectroscopy in adults: a work in progress. Anesth Analg 2012;115:1373–83.
67. Naidech AM, Bendok BR, Ault ML, et al. Monitoring with the Somanetics INVOS 5100C after aneurysmal subarachnoid hemorrhage. Neurocrit Care 2008;9: 326–31.
68. Gopinath SP, Robertson CS, Contant CF, et al. Jugular venous desaturation and outcome after head injury. J Neurol Neurosurg Psychiatry 1994;57(6):717–23.
69. Le Roux P. Physiological monitoring of the severe traumatic brain injury patient in the intensive care unit. Curr Neurol Neurosci Rep 2013;13(3):331.
70. Wartenberg KE, Schmidt JM, Mayer SA. Multimodality monitoring in neurocritical care. Crit Care Clin 2007;23:507–38.
71. de Lima Oliveira M, Kairalla AC, Fonoff ET, et al. Cerebral microdialysis in traumatic brain injury and subarachnoid hemorrhage: state of the art. Neurocrit Care 2013. [Epub ahead of print].
72. Bellander BM, Cantais E, Enblad P, et al. Consensus meeting on microdialysis in neurointensive care. Intensive Care Med 2004;30(12):2166–9.
73. Andrews PJ, Citerio G, Longhi L, et al. NICEM consensus on neurological monitoring in acute neurological disease. Intensive Care Med 2008;34:1362–70.
74. Mollaret P, Goulon M. Le coma dépassé (mémoire préliminaire). Rev Neurol (Paris) 1959;101:3–5.
75. Wijdicks E. The neurologist and Harvard criteria for brain death. Neurology 2003;61:970–6.
76. A definition of irreversible coma. Report of the Ad Hoc Committee of the Harvard Medical School to examine the definition of brain death. JAMA 1968;205:337–40.
77. Diagnosis of brain death. Statement issued by the honorary secretary of the Conference of Medical Royal Colleges and their Faculties in the United Kingdom on 11 October 1976. Br Med J 1976;2:1187–8.

78. Guidelines for the determination of death. Report of the medical consultants on the diagnosis of death to the President's Commission for the Study of Ethical Problems in Medicine and Biomedical and Behavioral Research. J Am Med Assoc 1981;248:2184–6.

79. Practice parameters for determining brain death in adults (summary statement). The Quality Standards Subcommittee of the American Academy of Neurology. Neurology 1995;45:1012–4.

80. Greer DM, Varelas PN, Haque S, et al. Variability of brain death determination guidelines in leading US neurologic institutions. Neurology 2008;70:284–9.

81. Wijdicks EF. Brain death worldwide: accepted fact but no global consensus in diagnostic criteria. Neurology 2002;58:20–5.

82. Schewmon DA. Brain death: can it be resuscitated? Hastings Cent Rep 2009; 39(2):18–24.

83. Safar P. Ventilatory efficacy of mouth-to-mouth artificial respiration: airway obstruction during manual and mouth-to-mouth artificial respiration. J Am Med Assoc 1958;167:335–41.

84. Kouwenhoven WB, Jude JR, Knickerbocker GG. Closed-chest cardiac massage. J Am Med Assoc 1960;173:1064–7.

85. Baskett PJ. The resuscitation greats: Peter J. Safar, the early years 1924-1961, the birth of CPR. Resuscitation 2001;50:17–22.

86. Williams GR, Spencer FC. The clinical use of hypothermia following cardiac arrest. Ann Surg 1958;148:462–5.

87. Hypothermia after Cardiac Arrest Study Group. Mild therapeutic hypothermia to improve the neurologic outcome after cardiac arrest. N Engl J Med 2002;346: 549–56.

88. Bernard SA, Gray TW, Buist MD, et al. Treatment of comatose survivors of out-of-hospital cardiac arrest with induced hypothermia. N Engl J Med 2002;346: 557–63.

89. Peberdy MA, Callaway CQ, Neumar RW, et al. Part 9: post cardiac arrest care: 2010 American Heart Association guidelines for cardiopulmonary resuscitation and emergency cardiovascular care. Circulation 2010;122:S768–86.

90. Hemphill JC, Andrews P, De Georgia M. Multimodal monitoring and neurocritical care bioinformatics. Nat Rev Neurol 2011;7:451–60.

91. Christophe M, Nicolas S. Mitochondria: a target for neuroprotective interventions in cerebral ischemia-reperfusion. Curr Pharm Des 2006;12(6):739–57.

92. Qureshi AI, Palesch YY. Antihypertensive treatment of acute cerebral hemorrhage (ATACH) II: design, methods, and rationale. Neurocrit Care 2011;15(3):559–76.

93. Tissue plasminogen activator for acute ischemic stroke. The National Institute of Neurological Disorders and Stroke rt-PA Stroke Study Group. N Engl J Med 1995;333:1581–7.

94. Mokin M, Khalessi AA, Mocco J, et al. Endovascular treatment of acute ischemic stroke: the end or just the beginning? Neurosurg Focus 2014;36(1):E5.

95. Winer JB. An update in Guillain-Barré syndrome. Autoimmune Dis 2014;2014: 793024.

96. Fisher M. An unusual variant of acute idiopathic polyneuritis: syndrome of ophtalmoplegia, ataxia and areflexia. N Engl J Med 1956;255:57–65.

97. Bickerstaff ER. Brain-stem encephalitis: further observations on a grave syndrome with benign prognosis. Br Med J 1957;1:1384–7.

98. Ito M, Kuwabara S, Odaka M, et al. Bickerstaff's brainstem encephalitis and Fisher syndrome form a continuous spectrum: clinical analysis of 581 cases. J Neurol 2008;255:674–82.

99. Graus F, Dalmau J. Paraneoplastic neurological syndromes. Curr Opin Neurol 2012;25(6):795–801.
100. Dalmau J, Tüzün E, Wu HY, et al. Paraneoplastic Anti-N-methyl-D-aspartate receptor encephalitis associated with ovarian teratoma. Ann Neurol 2007;61(1): 25–36.
101. Rincon F, Mayer SA. Neurocritical care: a distinct discipline? Curr Opin Crit Care 2007;13:115–21.
102. Suarez JI. Outcome in neurocritical care: advances in monitoring and treatment and effect of a specialized neurocritical care team. Crit Care Med 2006;34(9 Suppl):S232–8.
103. Mirski MA, Chang CW, Cowan R. Impact of a neuroscience intensive care unit on neurosurgical patient outcomes and cost of care: evidence-based support for an intensivist-directed specialty ICU model of care. J Neurosurg Anesthesiol 2001;13(2):83–92.

Update in the Management of Acute Ischemic Stroke

Nelson J. Maldonado, MD, Syed O. Kazmi, MD, Jose Ignacio Suarez, MD*

KEYWORDS

- Acute ischemic stroke • Thrombolysis • Hemicraniectomy • Critical care
- Neurocritical care • Outcomes • Neuroprotection • Cerebral edema

KEY POINTS

- All patients with acute ischemic stroke presenting within 4.5 hours of symptom onset must be considered for thrombolytic therapy. The sooner intravenous thrombolysis is administered, the better the outcome.
- Careful attention to blood pressure control is necessary. For patients receiving thrombolytic therapy, blood pressure should be kept lower than 180/105 mm Hg at all times within the first 24 hours.
- Patients with acute ischemic stroke requiring mechanical ventilation should be intubated using rapid sequence intubation while avoiding hypotension.
- Young patients presenting with severe strokes involving the middle cerebral artery territory should be considered for early decompressive hemicraniectomy to decrease mortality and improve functional outcome.
- All patients with acute ischemic stroke should be evaluated emergently and transported to specialized stroke centers to receive the best available care.

INTRODUCTION

Stroke is a common neurologic emergency and an important cause of death and disability in the United States. According to American Heart Association (AHA) statistics, approximately 795,000 Americans each year suffer a new or recurrent stroke, and approximately 137,000 of them will die.[1] Fortunately, overall evaluation, management, and outcome of patients with ischemic stroke have improved significantly. For example, stroke is currently the fourth cause of death in the United States, down from number 3 a few years ago. Much of this is due to the advent of thrombolytic therapy and the development of stroke systems of care, which have changed the way

Disclosures: None.
Division of Vascular Neurology and Neurocritical Care, Department of Neurology, Baylor College of Medicine, One Baylor Plaza, MS NB302, Houston, TX 77030, USA
* Corresponding author.
E-mail address: jisuarez@bcm.edu

http://dx.doi.org/10.1016/j.ccc.2014.06.002
0749-0704/14/$ – see front matter © 2014 Elsevier Inc. All rights reserved.
criticalcare.theclinics.com

practitioners view and treat this devastating disease.[2,3] Tools developed to improve early detection and increase potential for treatment include (1) the Newcastle face, arm, speech test (FAST) stroke warning sign and symptoms directed to educate the general population; (2) the Cincinnati prehospital stroke scale directed to emergency medical services (EMS) personnel; and (3) the stroke Chain of Survival directed to the EMS, emergency department (ED), and hospital stroke teams. The overall goal of these tools is to improve response time and care of patients with stroke and thus increase the number of patients receiving comprehensive treatments, including thrombolytic therapy, critical care, and rehabilitation.

In this review, we present an update on the management of acute ischemic stroke divided into the first 24 hours and then beyond with pertinent measures for the intensive care unit (ICU) setting. While discussing management within the initial 24 hours, we further differentiate between patients who receive recombinant tissue plasminogen activator (rt-PA) and patients who do not, as management differs between these 2 groups. Beyond the first 24 hours, the management of the patient with ischemic stroke is usually the same regardless of initial thrombolytic therapy.

INITIAL 24 HOURS FOR PATIENTS ELIGIBLE FOR THROMBOLYTIC THERAPY

The ultimate goal in the early management of acute ischemic stroke is to be able to administer thrombolytic therapy to all eligible patients in a timely manner. The benefit of this therapy is time dependent, TIME is BRAIN.

The initial evaluation of a patients with potential stroke starts with immediate stabilization of the airway, breathing, and circulation, which is usually performed by first responders (**Table 1**). Subsequently, patients should be transferred to hospitals or patient care areas appropriately staffed and equipped with dedicated stroke teams, stroke units, and neurocritical care expertise, as this has been shown to improve outcomes in terms of reduced death and disability rates compared with conventional care.[2,3]

Once in the ED, an initial clinical assessment remains the main tool for an accurate diagnosis of stroke. A brief patient history, including the determination of the time of symptom onset (last time the patient was seen normal), comorbidities, and medications will determine eligibility for thrombolytic therapy. The physical examination should be divided into a general and neurologic examination. Such examinations will help rule out other etiologies that can mimic stroke, such as trauma, infection, psychiatric disorders, and other systemic abnormalities.

The use of a stroke rating scale, such as the NIHSS (National Institutes of Health Stroke Scale), which is considered an abbreviated neurologic examination, has been developed as a tool to assess initial stroke symptoms, stroke severity, and guide management decisions before and after thrombolytic therapy.[4,5] Very importantly, the NIHSS should serve as a communication tool among ED physicians, neurologists, intensivists, and other health care personnel. The NIHSS can be used as a monitoring tool of progression or worsening throughout the patient in-hospital stay (**Table 2**). In addition, the Glasgow Coma Scale (GCS) can help monitor the level of consciousness and can guide in decisions regarding institution of mechanical ventilation, as will be discussed later (see **Table 2**).

After the initial physical examination is performed, the only tests that should always precede the decision to administer rt-PA in eligible patients are a noncontrast enhanced computed tomography (CT) scan of the brain, to rule out intracranial hemorrhage (absolute contraindication) (**Fig. 1**), and serum glucose (point-of-care testing) to evaluate for severe hyperglycemia or hypoglycemia. Other testing, such as hematologic workup, metabolic panel, coagulation tests, baseline troponins, and electrocardiogram (ECG), are recommended but should not delay the initiation of thrombolytic therapy.

Intravenous Thrombolytics

Intravenous (IV) rt-PA is currently the only treatment approved by the Food and Drug Administration (FDA) for acute ischemic stroke within the first few hours of symptom onset. In 1995, the National Institute of Neurologic Disorders rt-PA Stroke Study Group published a landmark study in acute stroke treatment.[4] The investigators showed that patients treated with rt-PA within 3 hours of symptom onset had a substantially better chance of functional independence with minimal or no disability 3 months after treatment with a single IV dose (0.9 mg/kg, maximum dose 90 mg). More recently, the European Cooperative Acute Stroke Study III trial showed that it was safe and still beneficial to increase the time window from symptom onset from 3.0 to 4.5 hours on selected patients (**Box 1**).[5]

It is crucial to understand that the benefit of thrombolytic therapy is time dependent and treatment should be initiated as quickly as possible. A pooled analysis from 4 of the most relevant IV rt-PA studies demonstrated that treatment within the first 90 minutes of onset increased the odds of an excellent outcome by 2.6-fold, in the 91-minute to 180-minute window by 1.6-fold, and in the 181-minute to 270-minute window by 1.3-fold.[6]

Despite this evidence, very few stroke patients are being treated with thrombolytic therapy in the United States. The AHA has been active at increasing awareness and enhancing treatment rates for this patient population. Currently the AHA acute stroke management guidelines recommend a door to needle time (bolus administration) of 60 minutes or less from hospital arrival.[7]

In patients without recent use of oral anticoagulants or heparin, treatment with IV rt-PA can be initiated before availability of coagulation test results but the infusion should be discontinued if the international normalized ratio (INR) is greater than 1.7 or prothrombin time is abnormally elevated by local laboratory standards.

In patients without history of thrombocytopenia, treatment with IV rt-PA can be initiated before availability of platelet count but should be discontinued if platelet count is less than 100,000/mm^3.

Antiplatelets and Anticoagulants

Antiplatelet and anticoagulant medications are not recommended for the first 24 hours after patients have received thrombolytic therapy. There is evidence that patients who receive aspirin within this time frame are at increased risk of hemorrhagic transformation.[8]

If IV anticoagulation is considered after 24 hours of thrombolysis administration, a noncontrast head CT scan or other sensitive diagnostic imaging method should be performed to rule out any intracranial hemorrhage before initiating this treatment.

Blood Pressure Management

Blood pressure (BP) monitoring and management is another important measure in the acute phase of ischemic stroke. BP needs to be closely monitored for the first 24 hours after thrombolytic therapy: initially every 15 minutes for 2 hours after starting the infusion, then every 30 minutes for 6 hours, and last every hour for 18 hours.

Before initiation of IV rt-PA in an eligible patient, the BP must be kept below 185/110 mm Hg and once the treatment is given it must be maintained below 180/105 mm Hg at all times for the first 24 hours. Current recommendations for BP

Table 1
Summary of key treatment modalities for patients with acute ischemic stroke

Intervention	Eligible for Thrombolysis	Not Eligible for Thrombolysis
First 24 h from symptom onset		
Initial evaluation	Airway, Breathing, and Circulation; NIHSS; GCS	
Airway protection with rapid sequence intubation	Etomidate 0.2–0.3 mg/kg IV; lidocaine 1–2 mg/kg IV; rocuronium 0.6–1.2 mg/kg IV	
Blood pressure control	Maintain <180/105 mm Hg; Use labetalol 10–20 mg IV over 1–2 min, may repeat; or nicardipine 5–15 mg/h; Avoid hypotension	Maintain <220/120 mm Hg; Use labetalol 10–20 mg IV over 1–2 min, may repeat; or nicardipine 5–15 mg/h; Avoid hypotension
IV fluids	0.9% saline	
Dysphagia screening	Yes; before any medications or food is given	
Antiplatelets	None	Aspirin 81–325 mg/d orally or clopidogrel 75 mg/d orally
DVT prophylaxis	Mechanical devices only	Low-molecular weight heparin (preferred) or unfractionated heparin
GI prophylaxis	H2-receptor blockers or proton-pump inhibitor	
Temperature	Maintain core body temperature <37.2°C; use acetaminophen and/or ibuprofen; refractory cases use external cooling devices	
Blood glucose	Maintain 140–180 mg/dL	
Statins	Yes; several options; high dose preferred	
Beyond 24 h from symptom onset		
Airway protection with rapid sequence intubation	Etomidate 0.2–0.3 mg/kg IV; lidocaine 1–2 mg/kg IV; rocuronium 0.6–1.2 mg/kg IV	

IV fluids	0.9% saline
Blood pressure control	Reasonable to initiate long-term antihypertensives; reduction 15%–20% of initial value
Management of cerebral edema	Head elevation 30°–45°; mannitol 1.0–1.5 g/kg IV bolus and subsequent doses of 0.25–1.0 g/kg, discontinue if serum osmolarity >325 mOsm/L or serum sodium >155 mEq/L; hypertonic saline: 3% saline (250–300 mL IV bolus) or 23.4% saline (30 mL IV bolus), both require central line; induced hyperventilation (keep $Paco_2$ 30–35 mm Hg) and wean as soon as feasible in increments of 1–2 breaths/min; sedation and analgesia
Temperature	Maintain core body temperature <37.2°C; use acetaminophen and/or ibuprofen; refractory cases use external cooling devices
Blood glucose	Maintain 140–180 mg/dL
DVT prophylaxis	Low-molecular weight heparin (preferred) or unfractionated heparin
GI prophylaxis	H2-receptor blockers or proton-pump inhibitor
Statins	Yes; several options; high dose preferred
Antiplatelets	Aspirin 81–325 mg/d orally or clopidogrel 75 mg/d orally
Oral anticoagulants	If cardioembolic source confirmed or suspected: warfarin (any atrial fibrillation); direct-thrombin and activated factor X inhibitors (nonvalvular atrial fibrillation)
CEA	Early CEA for patients with small, nondisabling strokes and large territory at risk, and stable neurologic examination
Decompressive craniectomy	Age 18–60 y; <45 h from symptom onset; NIHSS >15; >50% involvement of MCA territory by head imaging; should be performed as early as possible and before neurologic deterioration
Hemorrhagic transformation	Discontinue thrombolytics or anticoagulants immediately; administer cryoprecipitate, fresh-frozen plasma; consider platelet transfusion and prothrombin complex concentrate; neurosurgical evaluation

Abbreviations: CEA, carotid endarterectomy; DVT, deep venous thrombosis; GCS, Glasgow Coma Scale; GI, gastrointestinal; IV, intravenous; MCA, middle cerebral artery; NIHSS, National Institutes of Health stroke scale.

Table 2
National Institutes of Health Stroke Scale (NIHSS) and Glasgow Coma Scale (GCS)

NIHSS (range: 0–42 points): >15 indicates severe stroke; and increase ≥4 points indicates neurologic deterioration	GCS (range: 3–15): a decrease by ≥2 points indicates neurologic deterioration
1A Level of consciousness 　0—Alert 　1—Drowsy 　2—Obtunded 　3—Coma/unresponsive **1B** Orientation questions (2) 　0—Answers both correctly 　1—Answers 1 correctly 　2—Answers neither correctly **1C** Response to commands (2) 　0—Performs both tasks correctly 　1—Performs 1 task correctly 　2—Performs neither Best gaze 　0—Normal horizontal movements 　1—Partial gaze palsy 　2—Forced deviation Visual 　0—No visual field defect 　1—Partial hemianopia 　2—Complete hemianopia 　3—Bilateral hemianopia Facial palsy 　0—Normal 　1—Minor facial weakness 　2—Partial facial weakness 　3—Complete unilateral palsy **Motor arm** a. Left b. Right 　　0—No drift 　　1—Drift before 10 s 　　2—Falls before 10 s 　　3—No effort against gravity 　　4—No movement 　　UN— Amputation **Motor leg** a. Left b. Right 　　0—No drift 　　1—Drift before 5 s 　　2—Falls before 5 s 　　3—No effort against gravity 　　4—No movement 　　UN— Amputation Limb ataxia 　0—No ataxia 　1—Ataxia in 1 limb 　2—Ataxia in 2 limbs 　UN— Amputation	Eye Opening Response • Spontaneous—open with blinking at baseline: 4 points • To verbal stimuli, command, speech: 3 points • To pain only (not applied to face): 2 points • No response: 1 point Verbal Response • Oriented: 5 points • Confused conversation, but able to answer questions: 4 points • Inappropriate words: 3 points • Incomprehensible speech: 2 points • No response: 1 point Motor Response • Obeys commands for movement: 6 points • Purposeful movement to painful stimulus: 5 points • Withdraws in response to pain: 4 points • Flexion in response to pain (decorticate posturing): 3 points • Extension response in response to pain (decerebrate posturing): 2 points • No response: 1 point

Sensory
  0—No sensory loss
  1—Mild sensory loss
  2—Severe sensory loss
Best language
  0—Normal
  1—Mild aphasia
  2—Severe aphasia
  3—Mute or global aphasia
Articulation
  0—Normal
  1—Mild dysarthria
  2—Severe dysarthria
  UN— Intubated
Extinction or inattention
  0—Absent
  1—Mild (loss 1 sensory modality lost)
  2—Severe (loss 2 modalities lost)

elevation include IV boluses of labetalol 10 to 20 mg or an IV drip of nicardipine 5 to 15 mg/h.[5,7]

Early Imaging

The purpose of performing brain imaging is to confirm clinical suspicion of stroke, and to differentiate brain ischemia from hemorrhage, which is indispensable information before administration of thrombolytic therapy. Brain imaging will define the size and vascular distribution of ischemic stroke, which may influence immediate and long-term treatment decisions (see **Fig. 1**).

The most commonly used brain imaging modalities are CT and magnetic resonance imaging (MRI) (including diffusion-weighted imaging or DWI sequence). The latter has a better resolution and higher sensitivity and specificity to determine brain ischemia.[9] However, the imaging time for MRI is longer and is not available in all institutions.

Various advanced MRI and CT imaging techniques are available. However, to date there is no evidence that these advanced techniques are beneficial compared with plain head CT.[10] Non–contrast-enhanced CT scan remains sufficient for identification of contraindications to thrombolysis and must be obtained within 25 minutes of the patient's arrival in the ED.[7]

Several head CT scan findings have been reported in the acute phase of patients with ischemic stroke (see **Fig. 1**).[9,10] The most salient features include the following: loss of gray-white differentiation (lenticular obscuration or insular ribbon sign); swelling of the gyri that produces sulcal effacement; the hyperdense middle cerebral artery (MCA) sign, which represents an increased density within the occluded artery and possible large-vessel occlusion; hyperdense MCA "dot" sign, which may represent a clot within a branch of the MCA; and intracranial hemorrhage, which is an absolute contraindication for IV thrombolysis as mentioned previously.

A noninvasive evaluation of the intracranial and extracranial vessels is often performed in patients considered candidates for endovascular treatment (see later in this article). Such studies include magnetic resonance angiogram (MRA) or CT angiography (CTA) and can help screen patients with major vessel occlusions. However, these studies should not delay IV rt-PA administration. Further imaging, needed to clarify stroke etiology, can be done during the subsequent 24 hours. These include brain MRI or vessel studies, such as carotid ultrasound, transcranial Doppler

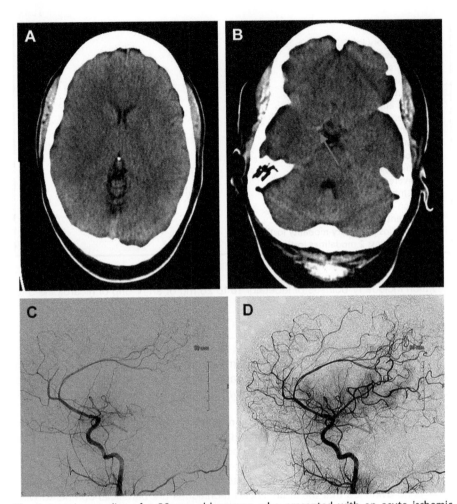

Fig. 1. Imaging studies of a 36-year-old woman who presented with an acute ischemic stroke involving her right MCA territory and NIHSS of 18. (*A*) Baseline head CT within 3 hours of symptom onset showed loss of gray-white matter differentiation in the right MCA territory and sulcal effacement. (*B*) Hyperdense right MCA sign is seen (*arrow*). (*C*) After IV thrombolysis, patient was taken to cerebral angiogram, which showed complete occlusion of right MCA (*arrow*). (*D*) Patient underwent endovascular therapy and a follow-up cerebral angiogram showed recanalization of occluded right MCA (*arrows*). (*E*) MRI of her brain showing a large right MCA territory infarction (DWI). (*F*) A follow-up head CT scan 24 hours later showed right hemispheric edema with some midline shift. (*G*) Patient underwent right decompressive hemicraniectomy as shown on the head CT scan. (*H*) Patient was discharged to rehabilitation and 6 weeks later underwent right cranioplasty as shown on head CT scan. She returned to clinic 3 months later ambulating with a cane.

ultrasound, CTA, and MRA. If there is concern for acute medical deterioration, then a repeat emergent head CT scan or brain MRI should be considered to evaluate for hemorrhagic conversion, recurrent strokes, or cerebral edema. It is also recommended to perform a follow-up head CT scan in all patients after 24 hours of IV rt-PA administration to rule out hemorrhagic conversion.

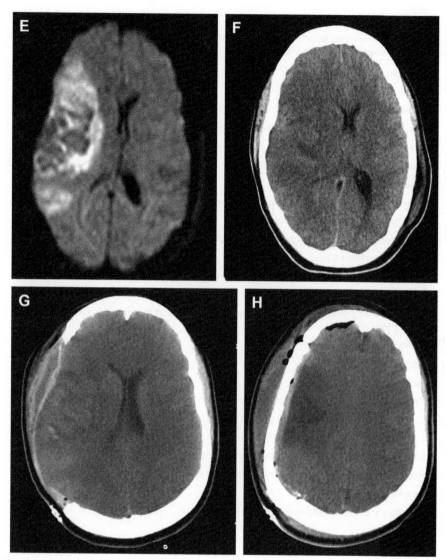

Fig. 1. (*continued*)

Other Testing

There are other diagnostic tests that can be performed acutely in the evaluation of ischemic stroke (**Box 2**).[7] Some of these diagnostic evaluations should be performed in all patients, such as basic serum laboratory testing, ECG, and determination of arterial oxygen saturation (SaO$_2$). However, many of these are optional and should be performed in selected patients and depending on specific circumstances.

Endovascular Management

There has been much advancement in endovascular management for treatment of acute ischemic stroke. This includes endovascular pharmacologic thrombolysis, manipulation of

Box 1
Inclusion and exclusion criteria for patients with acute ischemic stroke for IV thrombolysis within 4.5 hours of symptom onset

Within 3 hours of symptom onset

Inclusion criteria

    Measurable neurologic deficit (abnormal NIHSS) due to ischemic stroke

    Clear onset of symptoms <3 hours before beginning treatment

    Aged ≥18 years

    Head CT scan without ICH

Exclusion criteria

    Severe head trauma or prior stroke in previous 3 months

    Suspicion of subarachnoid hemorrhage

    Arterial puncture at noncompressible site in previous 7 days

    History of previous ICH

    Intracranial neoplasm, arteriovenous malformation, or aneurysm

    Recent intracranial or intraspinal surgery

    Elevated blood pressure (systolic >185 mm Hg or diastolic >110 mm Hg) not responsive to IV medications

    Active systemic bleeding

    Acute bleeding diathesis

    Platelet count <100,000/mm^3

    Heparin received within 48 hours, resulting in abnormally elevated aPTT

    Current use of warfarin with INR greater than 1.7 or PT greater than 15 seconds

    Current use of direct thrombin inhibitors or direct factor Xa inhibitors

    Blood glucose concentration less than 50 mg/dL (2.7 mmol/L)

    Head CT demonstrates hypodensity greater than one-third cerebral hemisphere

Relative exclusion criteria

    Only minor or rapidly improving stroke symptoms

    Pregnancy

    Seizure at onset with postictal neurologic impairments

    Major surgery or serious trauma within previous 14 days

    Recent gastrointestinal or urinary tract hemorrhage (within previous 21 days)

    Acute myocardial infarction within previous 3 months

From 3 to 4.5 hours of symptom onset

Inclusion criteria

    Measurable neurologic deficit (abnormal NIHSS) due to ischemic stroke

    Clear onset of symptoms 3–4.5 hours before beginning treatment

    Aged ≥18 years

    Head CT scan without ICH

Relative exclusion criteria

Aged older than 80 years

Severe stroke (NIHSS>25)

Taking an oral anticoagulant regardless of INR

History of both diabetes and prior ischemic stroke

Abbreviations: aPTT, activated thromboplastin time; CT, computed tomography; ICH, intracranial hemorrhage; INR, international normalized ratio; IV, intravenous; NIHSS, National Institutes of Health stroke scale.

Data from The National Institute of Neurological Disorders and Stroke rt-PA Study Group. Tissue plasminogen activator for acute ischemic stroke. N Engl J Med 1995;333:1581–7; and Hacke W, Kaste M, Bluhmki E, et al. Thrombolysis with alteplase 3 to 4.5 hours after acute ischemic stroke. N Engl J Med 2008;359:1317–29.

the clot using a guidewire or microcatheter, mechanical and aspiration thrombectomy, and stent retriever technology.[11] These techniques theoretically allow better recanalization of the occluded vessel albeit at the expense of valuable time. The Prolyse in Acute Cerebral Thromboembolism II trial[12] of recombinant prourokinase (r-pro-UK) was published in 1999 and showed that intra-arterial (IA) use of r-pro-UK within 6 hours of stroke symptom onset achieved MCA recanalization in 66% of the treated arm compared with 18% in the control

Box 2
Current recommendations and practice regarding ancillary testing in patients with acute ischemic stroke

ALL patients

- Blood glucose (point-of-care or laboratory testing)
- SaO_2
- Serum electrolytes and creatinine
- Complete blood count
- Serum troponin levels
- PT/INR and aPTT
- ECG

SELECTED patients (to be decided on individual patients)

- TT and/or ECT if patient is taking direct thrombin inhibitors or direct factor Xa inhibitors
- Liver function tests
- Toxicology screen and blood alcohol level
- Pregnancy test
- Chest radiography
- Electroencephalogram
- Echocardiogram

Abbreviations: aPTT, activated thromboplastin time; ECG, electrocardiogram; ECT, ecarin time; INR, international normalized ratio; PT, prothrombin time; SaO_2, arterial oxygen saturation; TT, thrombin time.

Data from Refs.[4,5,7,11,34]

group. This IA approach, which was extrapolated to rt-PA, is thought to be more efficacious for proximal arterial occlusions.[13] Hence, large proximal thrombi of a major intracranial vessel in patients ineligible for intravenous rt-PA has been considered an indication for IA thrombolysis. However, the optimal dose of IA rt-PA is not well established, and has not been approved by the FDA.[14]

Endovascular techniques, such as the mechanical embolus removal in cerebral ischemia (MERCI) retriever, Penumbra System, Solitaire FR revascularization technique, and the thrombectomy revascularization of large vessel occlusion (TREVO) retrieval system, have been shown to increase rates of recanalization either with or without intravenous rt-PA. The MERCI retriever was evaluated in patients ineligible for intravenous rt-PA and with arterial occlusions who presented within 8 hours of stroke symptom onset in the MERCI trial.[15] The Penumbra System was evaluated in a prospective study of patients with NIHSS scores of 8 or higher who presented within 8 hours of symptom onset.[16] The SWIFT study (Solitaire FR With the Intention for Thrombectomy)[17] and the TREVO 2 study[18] compared the Solitaire FR and TREVO devices with the MERCI Retrieval system, respectively. Both devices were independently deemed superior to the MERCI Retrieval system in achieving recanalization. Hence, when mechanical thrombectomy is pursued, stent retrievers, such as Solitaire FR and TREVO, are generally preferred to coil retrievers, such as MERCI.[7] The relative effectiveness of the Penumbra System versus stent retrievers has not yet been characterized. However, these devices have not been demonstrated to improve patient outcomes compared with IV rt-PA. The Interventional Management of Stroke III[11] trial and the Local versus Systemic Thrombolysis for Acute Ischemic Stroke[19] trial showed that there was no difference between endovascular treatment compared with standard IV rt-PA for acute ischemic stroke. The MR RESCUE (Mechanical Retrieval and Recanalization of Stroke Clots Using Embolectomy) trial was not able to identify a favorable penumbral pattern on neuroimaging that would benefit from endovascular therapy for acute ischemic stroke nor did it show embolectomy to be superior to standard of care.[20]

The usefulness of emergent intracranial or extracranial angioplasty/stenting has not been well established in the setting of acute ischemic stroke. With regard to intracranial atherosclerotic disease, the SAMMPRIS (Stenting and Aggressive Medical Management for Preventing Recurrent Stroke in Intracranial Stenosis) trial effectively proved that aggressive medical management was superior to percutaneous transluminal angioplasty and stenting in the subacute setting for patients with symptomatic intracranial stenosis.[21] Whether the SAMMPRIS trial results can be extrapolated to the management of acute ischemic stroke remains to be determined.

Dysphagia Screening

All patients should have an NPO (nothing by mouth) status at the time of hospital arrival and be screened for swallowing deficits before eating or drinking or taking oral medications.[7] The presence of a gag reflex is not a valid screen for dysphagia. If patients fail their swallowing evaluation, alternative ways of nutrition need to be implemented to decrease the risk of aspiration and to be able to provide adequate caloric intake as soon as possible.

INITIAL 24 HOURS FOR PATIENTS INELIGIBLE FOR THROMBOLYTIC THERAPY
Pharmacologic Strategies

Antiplatelet agents

Patients not eligible for IV rt-PA should be administered aspirin immediately. This can be given orally if the patient is able to swallow. Otherwise, aspirin should be given rectally. Two large randomized-controlled clinical trials demonstrated reduction in death and disability with aspirin when it was begun 48 hours after stroke onset.[22,23] The role of clopidogrel remains limited in the acute stroke setting. However, a recent randomized, controlled clinical trial demonstrated better protection with aspirin and clopidogrel for subsequent strokes compared with aspirin alone in the first 90 days without increasing the risk of intracranial hemorrhage (ICH).[24] The use of other anti-platelet agents, such as IV abciximab,[25–28] tirofiban,[29] and eptifibatide,[30] have been studied in the setting of acute stroke but are not yet recommended.

Anticoagulants/Antithrombotic agents

The use of anticoagulants in the setting of an acute ischemic stroke has been declining. Data on the administration of heparin and other anticoagulants in the emergent setting has been negative or inconclusive.[14,31–36] The optimal timing on the use of warfarin for patients with nonvalvular atrial fibrillation is unknown. However, it seems reasonable to initiate anticoagulation with a goal of reaching a therapeutic range within 7 to 14 days.[37,38] Newer antithrombotic agents, such as the direct thrombin inhibitor, dabigatran, and Factor Xa inhibitors, apixaban and rivaroxaban, have been shown to prevent recurrent stroke in patients with nonvalvular atrial fibrillation.

BP management

The threshold for BP management is 220/120 for patients who are ineligible for IV thrombolysis. This higher cutoff is due mainly in part to the theory of peri-infarct penumbral protection. Higher BP may result in hypertensive encephalopathy and worsening cerebral edema.[7] There have been multiple studies including randomized control trials looking at BP reduction in the setting of an acute ischemic stroke and outcomes.[39–43] The results of these studies have been inconclusive with no concrete evidence to support a precise BP parameter in the days following the ischemic insult. It is currently recommended to lower the BP no more than 15% within the first 24 hours after an ischemic stroke.[7]

Arterial hypotension has been associated with poor clinical outcomes and should be avoided.[43–46] The exact definition for arterial hypotension should be defined on an individual basis. Urgent correction of hypotension is mandated in all cases of cerebral ischemia, as this can worsen neurologic outcome. Use of vasopressors to reverse hypotension is considered reasonable if necessary.[7] The administration of high-dose albumin,[47] mechanical flow augmentation,[48,49] and induced hypertension[50–53] are not well established in the setting of acute ischemic stroke, and cannot be recommended at this time.

Deep venous thrombosis prophylaxis

Deep venous thrombosis (DVT) prophylaxis should be initiated on admission. DVT and associated pulmonary embolism (PE) account for significant morbidity and mortality after a stroke.[54] Low molecular weight heparin or heparinoid is more effective than unfractionated heparin in preventing DVT.[55,56] However, there is insufficient evidence to determine whether there is a difference for clinically important end points, such as symptomatic DVT/PE, ICH, major extracranial hemorrhage, and mortality.[56]

Temperature

Normothermia should be the goal for patients with acute ischemic stroke. Hyperthermia is associated with poor neurologic outcomes[57–59] with a twofold increased risk in short-term mortality in patients with acute stroke and hyperthermia within the first 24 hours of hospitalization. Even though hyperthermia may be secondary to the stroke that led to the hospitalization, other reasons must be considered first, such as infection, medications, and DVT. It is important to keep in mind that some infectious disorders like endocarditis are associated with fever and may be the cause of the stroke.

Once the workup and treatment of underlying causes of hyperthermia have been initiated, it is paramount to reduce the body temperature. The latter can be accomplished by either mechanical or pharmacologic means. The first line of treatment is acetaminophen, followed by ibuprofen and aspirin. There are no clinical trials available to determine whether medications are better than placebo in this setting. In patients who are refractory to medications, other measures, such as cooling devices, can be tried, but management of shivering may be necessary.[60]

Blood glucose control

Normoglycemia should be maintained after an acute ischemic stroke in the ICU. Hypoglycemia (blood glucose <60 mg/dL) should be treated, as this can result in permanent brain damage. Symptoms such as disorientation, dizziness, and slowing of speech have been noted with glucose levels drop below 47 mg/dL.[61,62] Treatment of hyperglycemia in an acute stroke was studied in the Glucose Insulin in Stroke Trial-UK with inconclusive results.[63] It is reasonable to maintain a blood glucose level within a range of 140 to 180 mg/dL in hospitalized patients following the recommendations from the AHA/American Stroke Association (ASA)[7] and American Dietetic Association recommendations until further data from randomized, controlled clinical trials become available.[64]

Gastrointestinal prophylaxis

Gastrointestinal (GI) hemorrhage after an acute ischemic stroke has been studied and can be a cause of mortality in the ICU setting.[65] ICU patients at risk for GI bleeding include those on mechanical ventilation, patients in a coma, patients receiving therapy with ulcerogenic drugs, and patients with prior GI bleeds.[66,67] Usually, GI bleeding in ICU patients is associated with erosive gastritis localized to the fundus and body of the stomach.[68] H2-recceptor blockers or proton pump inhibitors are the agents of choice for lesions that cause GI bleeding and should be used as prophylaxis.[69]

Because clopidogrel is a prodrug that requires conversion to its active metabolite, strong CYP2C19 inhibitors, such as omeprazole and esomeprazole will reduce its antiplatelet effect. The FDA prescribing information recommends avoiding concomitant administration of clopidogrel and these proton pump inhibitors.

Hydration and fluid status

Patients with acute stroke should be maintained euvolemic at all times in the ICU, preferably by administering isotonic crystalloids, such as 0.9% saline. Hypovolemia and dehydration should be avoided, as they can worsen cerebral ischemia. In addition, hypervolemia and the administration of hypotonic solutions should be avoided in patients with large strokes because of the risk of cerebral edema. The infusion of human albumin has not been shown to improve outcome in patients with acute stroke and is currently not recommended.[47]

Nonpharmacologic Strategies

Cardiac monitoring

Continuous cardiac monitoring, which is easily accomplished in the ICU setting, is indicated for at least the first 24 hours after symptom onset. This is not only to determine possible stroke etiology but also to monitor for possible acute arrhythmias secondary to stroke.[70–72] However, longer monitoring, such as prolonged Holter monitoring, has been demonstrated to be more effective in identifying atrial fibrillation or other arrhythmias after stroke.[73] Current 2014 AHA/ASA guidelines recommend prolonged rhythm monitoring for approximately 30 days within 6 months of the index event.[74]

MANAGEMENT OF ACUTE ISCHEMIC STROKE BEYOND THE INITIAL 24 HOURS

Patients with acute ischemic stroke remain at high risk of experiencing secondary brain damage and recurrent cerebral ischemia beyond the initial 24 hours of symptom onset whether they receive IV thrombolysis or not. Therefore, there is a need for ongoing close monitoring and management particularly if patients require ICU care (see **Table 1**). Several studies support the fact that admission to a specialized stroke unit significantly improves patients' outcomes by decreasing death and disability. Therefore, the availability of stroke unit care is one of the cornerstone recommendations for improving stroke management.[2,7,75–77] Furthermore, many of these patients become critically ill requiring ventilatory support or develop complications that require management in a neuro-ICU. The availability of a specialized neuro-ICU with care directed by a neurocritical care team is associated with reduction of mortality and overall improved outcomes of these patients.[78]

Pharmacologic Strategies

BP management

BP is initially increased then declines spontaneously within the first few days after stroke. It is very important to understand that after an ischemic stroke the cerebral autoregulatory mechanisms may become abnormal and fail, and in these instances the cerebral blood flow will become directly proportional to the mean BP. If the latter happens, then any drop in BP could potentially decrease the cerebral blood flow at the already ischemic/penumbra region, thereby increasing stroke size. On the other hand, excessively high BP may worsen outcomes as well. The recommended medications are the same and have been discussed previously.[7]

General management

Management of volume status, BP, glucose and temperature, and DVT and GI prophylaxis were discussed previously for the initial 24-hour management for patients who are not eligible for IV thrombolysis.[7] The same measures should apply for all patients beyond the first 24 hours of symptom onset (see **Table 1**).

Mixed Pharmacologic and Nonpharmacological Strategies

Airway management and mechanical ventilation

Approximately 10% of patients with acute ischemic stroke will experience respiratory failure requiring ventilatory support, and the frequency is usually much higher in those patients with significant MCA involvement.[79–82] The most common triggers for initiation of mechanical ventilation are decreased level of consciousness (defined as GCS <8) with concern for airway protection, elective intubation before procedures, and management of elevated intracranial pressure (ICP) and cerebral edema. Other indications for mechanical ventilation include respiratory and cardiac decompensation including hypoxemia (Pa_{O_2} <60 mm Hg), hypercarbia (Pa_{CO_2} >60 mm Hg), pulmonary edema, and tachypnea (respiratory rate >35/min) with use of accessory muscles.

Acute rises in ICP, hypertension, and hypotension are the most feared consequences of endotracheal intubation. Therefore, it is recommended that rapid sequence intubation (RSI) techniques are used and that medications that minimize complications are chosen.[83–85] Classic RSI involves successive administration of a rapid-acting induction agent and neuromuscular blocking agent.[86] Previous practice of applying cricoid pressure via the Sellick maneuver is currently controversial as to whether it effectively prevents aspiration.[87] Preferred IV medications include etomidate (0.2–0.3 mg/kg), which provides short-term sedation without significantly lowering the BP; lidocaine (1–2 mg/kg), which blunts the cough reflex preventing subsequent dangerous rises in ICP; and rocuronium (0.6–1.2 mg/kg), which provides muscle paralysis without affecting ICP. Depolarizing neuromuscular blockading agent succinylcholine (1–2 mg/kg) is sometimes used instead of rocuronium because of its shorter half-life. However, it has been associated with ICP elevations and hyperkalemia in neurologic patients. Once patients are mechanically ventilated, it is important to administer sedation for comfort and to avoid BP and ICP fluctuations. Sedation after intubation in neurologic patients is often achieved by shorter-acting medications, such as fentanyl, propofol, or midazolam.

There are no randomized-controlled clinical trials investigating various modes of ventilation and strategies in patients with acute ischemic stroke. Especially when ICP is a concern in patients with large stroke, to maintain a fixed minute ventilation, volume control is the most commonly used mode of ventilation. The main goals of mechanical ventilation are to maintain adequate oxygenation (SaO_2 >92%), and CO2 ($Paco_2$ between 35 and 45 mm Hg) levels without causing lung injury. Lung-protective ventilation should be undertaken whenever possible.[88,89] Such ventilatory strategy includes ventilation with a lower tidal volume, which involves an initial tidal volume of 6 to 8 mL per kilogram of predicted body weight, positive end-expiratory positive pressure of 5 cm H_2O, and a plateau pressure of 30 cm of water or less. However, tight monitoring of $Paco_2$ is mandatory, as a side effect of this therapy is hypercarbia. Significant changes in $Paco_2$ either toward high or low levels will affect the cerebral vasculature autoregulation capabilities, which can be deleterious to the already injured brain tissue.

Weaning from mechanical ventilation should be carried out in a fashion similar to other patients in the ICU.[89] The main criteria for weaning and trial of extubation include the following: improvement or correction of underlying disease, adequate oxygenation (SaO_2 >92% with Fio_2 <50%), adequate ventilation, hemodynamic instability (no hypotension or minimal vasopressor support), rapid shallow breathing index less than 105, absence of major electrolyte abnormalities, and adequate airway protection. The latter is usually the main impediment to extubation in this patient population as patients frequently have poor gag reflexes and may have injury to the lower brainstem, along with prolonged alteration of level of consciousness. Whether early tracheostomy improves outcome remains to be determined. However, a common practice is to perform early tracheostomies in patients with large MCA and posterior fossa strokes.

Acute neurologic worsening

Acute neurologic worsening can be defined as an increase in the NIHSS by more than 4 points or a decrease in the GCS by more than 2 points.[4,5,7] Approximately 25% of patients with acute stroke will experience neurologic deterioration within the first few days after symptom onset. The most common reasons for neurologic deterioration are cerebral edema, hemorrhagic transformation, stroke progression, recurrent stroke, and seizures.

Cerebral edema Infarcted brain matter swells, which in turn can lead to compression of surrounding structures and ultimately to tissue shifts and elevated ICP.[90–93] The latter usually occurs late and after tissue shifts and clinical signs of herniation have developed.[90] Therefore, ICP monitoring is rarely performed in this setting. The conditions in which cerebral edema occur after ischemic stroke are not fully clarified, but it is believed that tissue hypoxia and neuronal cell death will trigger the process. Cerebral edema will occur in all strokes. However, the degree of neurologic complications that cerebral edema can produce will vary from asymptomatic to life-threatening, depending on several factors, such as stroke size and location (MCA and cerebellar strokes), patients' age (younger patients are at higher risk), and preexisting level of brain atrophy.[90–94] Cytotoxic edema will usually peak between days 3 and 4 after stroke; however, some patients can develop brain edema within the first 24 hours, known as malignant edema, specifically large MCA and cerebellar infarctions.[91,93,94]

Careful observation in the ICU is required for patients at risk of significant edema. In general, the factors associated with life-threatening edema include the following: NIHSS greater than 15; greater than 50% hypodensity in the MCA territory, complete posterior inferior cerebellar artery (PICA), or superior cerebellar artery (SCA) territories on head CT scan; effacement of the basal cisterns, displacement of the pineal gland or brainstem, and hydrocephalus on head CT scan.[90–94] Clinical signs of brain tissue shift and herniation include a decrease in GCS greater than 2 points, unilaterally dilated or poorly responsive pupils, and extensor posturing.

Several medical interventions have been used to treat cerebral edema and herniation. These interventions are similar to those used in other neurocritical care conditions associated with cerebral edema.[92,93,95–97] Positioning of the patient with head elevation of 30 to 45° will improve cerebral venous drainage and any agent that causes cerebral vasodilation should be avoided. In addition, strategies such as controlled hyperventilation, sedation and analgesia, hypertonic agents, osmotic diuretics, cerebrospinal fluid diversion, and decompressive surgery can be done depending on ICP and edema severity (see **Table 1**).

Seizures The frequency of seizures in patients with acute ischemic stroke has been reported at approximately 10%, but may be higher in those with hemorrhagic transformation.[98,99] Patients should undergo immediate treatment as soon as seizures are suspected or encountered in a similar fashion as other neurologic patients (see **Table 1**).[100] There are no data supporting the administration of prophylactic antiepileptic drugs and as such should be avoided.

Surgical options

Endarterectomy There has been much controversy as to the role of early versus late carotid endarterectomy (CEA) for patients with ischemic strokes due to large vessel disease. Some investigators have justified early or even immediate surgical intervention on the basis of reducing the risk of recurrent strokes while waiting for revascularization.[101,102] On the other hand, there is a concern that CEA in the acute phase may cause hemorrhagic transformation of the ischemic infarct by hyperperfusion injury with a potential to increase cerebral edema. A systematic review was carried out on 47 studies to examine the optimal timing of CEA.[103] The investigators reported that there was a higher number of stroke and death rates with emergent CEA with no improvement in clinical status over time, especially in those patients with large disabling strokes with an unstable neurologic status. However, early CEA for carotid stenosis in small, nondisabling strokes with a higher vascular territory at risk and stable neurologic examination may be appropriate.[104–106] The most common indication for emergent surgical intervention is in the setting of a new neurologic deficit following a CEA to correct a technical issue that may have resulted in acute thrombosis.[7] Patients with a mobile or sessile intraluminal thrombus at the carotid bifurcation may benefit from emergent CEA, although better results have been reported with anticoagulation followed by delayed surgery.[107–110]

Decompressive craniectomy and external ventricular drain insertion Severe cerebral edema may not only lead to brainstem compression but also to compression of cerebral vessels, which can in turn produce cerebral infarctions.[91–93] This will further decrease the potential for meaningful clinical recovery in patients who survive these insults.

Earlier case series reports suggested that surgical decompression can reduce mortality from 80% to about 20% in patients with malignant MCA strokes.[91,92] However, it was unclear whether this surgical procedure was associated with improved functional outcome. Vahedi and colleagues[111] showed in a pooled analysis of 3 randomized controlled clinical trials that in a selective patient population, early decompressive hemicraniectomy with durotomy not only resulted in decreased mortality (79% in the surgery group vs 29% in the control group) but also improved functional outcome. Based on these results, decompressive hemicraniectomy with durotomy has become accepted as a modality of treatment for the following patients: age 18 to 60 years, surgical procedure within 45 hours of symptom onset and preferably before initiation of treatment for elevated ICP, NIHSS greater than 15, and evidence by imaging studies of greater than 50% involvement of the MCA territory. A more recent clinical trial evaluating decompressive hemicraniectomy in older stroke patients (61–82 years) also showed a significant reduction in mortality (70% in the surgery group vs 33% in the control group) with improvement in severe disability (38% vs 18%).[112] However, most survivors required assistance with most bodily needs. Due to these results, the decision to perform decompressive surgery should be made on an individual basis in older patients because of the potential undesired outcome of survival with severe disability.

Large strokes of the cerebellum (complete PICA and SCA territories) are usually associated with swelling in the posterior fossa, where the brainstem is located. Brainstem compression can be lethal, progression is usually rapid toward loss of brain stem functions. Decompressive suboccipital craniectomy and insertion of an external ventricular drain is often lifesaving if done early in the course of the stroke and is associated with improved quality of life in at least 50% of survivors.[113,114]

Hemorrhagic transformation The natural history of ischemic strokes shows that about 1% of patients can undergo spontaneous symptomatic hemorrhagic transformation. However, when thrombolytic therapy is administered, the rate of hemorrhagic transformation will increase to 6% to 10% depending on how early after the onset of stroke symptoms that IV rt-PA is given.[4–8]

Even though most hemorrhagic transformation will occur within the first 24 hours after IV rt-PA, we have included this subtopic here because of the potential for surgical intervention.[8] Once the possibility of ICH is suspected in patients with neurologic deterioration, prompt management is required. If symptoms of ICH present during the IV rt-PA infusion, then it should be stopped immediately and a noncontrast head CT scan should be obtained along with blood coagulation parameters, including type and screen and fibrinogen levels. Once ICH is confirmed, then coagulopathy reversal must be instituted immediately. There is no standardized and tested protocol for management of thrombolytic-associated ICH; however, most centers administer cryoprecipitate to restore fibrinogen levels to normal.[7,9] In addition, platelet infusion, fresh-frozen plasma, or prothrombin complex concentrates are also given because often these patients have abnormal platelet function and elevated INR.[115] Furthermore, a neurosurgical consultation should be sought. However, any neurosurgical procedure in this setting is performed as a life-saving maneuver and needs to be determined individually.

SUMMARY

Advances in the acute care of a patients with ischemic stroke, including the use of intravenous cerebral thrombolysis and intra-arterial catheter-based modalities for cerebrovascular disease, came of age around the same time that neurocritical care gained wider recognition as a subspecialty. Emergent therapy, followed by deliberate and thoughtful management at the bedside provided by dedicated stroke teams, stroke units, and neurocritical care expertise, can improve outcome. Practitioners continue to search for methods to deliver rapid care to patients who may benefit, while also evaluating the care given at the bedside to decrease complications and increase the chance for full functional outcome.

REFERENCES

1. Go AS, Mozaffarian D, Roger VL, et al. Executive summary: heart disease and stroke statistics-2014 update: a report from the American Heart Association. Circulation 2014;129:399–410.
2. Stroke Unit Trailists Collaboration. Organized inpatient (stroke unit) care for stroke. Cochrane Database Syst Rev 2007;(4):CD000197.
3. Govan L, Langhorne P, Weir CJ. Does the prevention of complications explain the survival benefit of organized impatient (stroke unit) care? Further analysis of a systematic review. Stroke 2007;38:2536–40.
4. The National Institute of Neurological Disorders and Stroke rt-PA Study Group. Tissue plasminogen activator for acute ischemic stroke. N Engl J Med 1995; 333:1581–7.
5. Hacke W, Kaste M, Bluhmki E, et al. Thrombolysis with alteplase 3 to 4.5 hours after acute ischemic stroke. N Engl J Med 2008;359:1317–29.
6. Lees KR, Bluhmki E, von Kummer R, et al. Time to treatment with intravenous alteplase and outcome in stroke: an updated pooled analysis of ECASS, ATLANTIS, NINDS, and EPITHET trials. Lancet 2010;375:1695–703.
7. Jauch EC, Saver JL, Adams HP Jr, et al. Guidelines for the early management of patients with acute ischemic stroke: a guideline for healthcare professionals from the American Heart Association/American Stroke Association. Stroke 2013;44:870–947.
8. Zinkstok SM, Roos YB, ARTIS Investigators. Early administration of aspirin in patients treated with alteplase for acute ischaemic stroke: a randomized controlled trial. Lancet 2012;380:731–7.
9. Brazzelli M, Sandercock PA, Chappell FM, et al. Magnetic resonance imaging versus computed tomography for the detection of acute vascular lesions in patients presenting with stroke symptoms. Cochrane Database Syst Rev 2009;(4):CD007424.
10. Wardlaw JM, Stevenson MD, Chapell F, et al. Carotid artery imaging for secondary stroke prevention: both imaging modality and rapid access to imaging are important. Stroke 2009;40:3511–7.
11. Broderick JP, Palesch YY, Demchuk AM, et al. Endovascular therapy after intravenous t-PA versus t-PA alone for stroke. N Engl J Med 2013;368:893–903.
12. Furlan A, Higashida R, Wechsler L, et al. Intra-arterial prourokinase for acute ischemic stroke: the PROACT II study: a randomized controlled trial: Prolyse in Acute Cerebral Thromboembolism. JAMA 1999;282:2003–11.
13. Mattle HP, Arnold M, Georgiadis D, et al. Comparison of intraarterial and intravenous thrombolysis for ischemic stroke with hyperdense middle cerebral artery sign. Stroke 2008;39:379–83.

14. Adams HP Jr, del Zoppo G, Alberts MJ, et al. Guidelines for the early management of adults with ischemic stroke: a guideline from the American Heart Association/American Stroke Association Stroke Council, Clinical Cardiology Council, Cardiovascular Radiology and Intervention Council, and the Atherosclerotic Peripheral Vascular Disease and Quality of Care Outcomes in Research Interdisciplinary Working Groups [Erratum in Stroke 2007;38:e38 and Stroke 2007;38:e96]. Stroke 2007;38:1655–711.

15. Smith WS, Sung G, Starkman S, et al. Safety and efficacy of mechanical embolectomy in acute ischemic stroke: results of the MERCI trial. Stroke 2005;36: 1432–8.

16. The Penumbra Pivotal Stroke Trial Investigators. The Penumbra Pivotal Stroke Trial: safety and effectiveness of a new generation of mechanical devices for clot removal in intracranial large vessel occlusive disease. Stroke 2009;40:2761–8.

17. Saver JL, Jahan R, Levy EI, et al. Solitaire flow restoration device versus the Merci Retriever in patients with acute ischaemic stroke (SWIFT): a randomised, parallel-group, non-inferiority trial. Lancet 2012;380:1241–9.

18. Nogueira RG, Lutsep HL, Gupta R, et al. Trevo versus Merci retrievers for thrombectomy revascularisation of large vessel occlusions in acute ischaemic stroke (TREVO 2): a randomized trial [Erratum appears in Lancet 2012;380:1230]. Lancet 2012;380:1231–40.

19. Ciccone A, Valvassori L, Nichelatti M, et al. Endovascular treatment for acute ischemic stroke. N Engl J Med 2013;368:904–13.

20. Kidwell CS, Jahan R, Gornbein J, et al. A trial of imaging selection and endovascular treatment for acute ischemic stroke. N Engl J Med 2013;368:914–23.

21. Chimowitz MI, Lynn MJ, Derdeyn CP, et al. Stenting versus aggressive medical therapy for intracranial arterial stenosis. N Engl J Med 2011;365:993–1003.

22. CAST (Chinese Acute Stroke Trial) Collaborative Group. CAST: randomized placebo-controlled trial of early aspirin use in 20,000 patients with acute ischaemic stroke. Lancet 1997;349:1641–9.

23. International Stroke Trial Collaborative Group. The International Stroke Trial (IST): a randomised trial of aspirin, subcutaneous heparin, both, or neither among 19435 patients with acute ischaemic stroke. Lancet 1997;349:1569–81.

24. Wang Y, Wang Y, Zhao X, et al. Clopidogrel with aspirin in acute minor stroke or transient ischemic attack. N Engl J Med 2013;369:11–9.

25. The Abciximab in Ischemic Stroke Investigators. Abciximab in acute ischemic stroke: a randomized, double-blind, placebo-controlled, dose-escalation study. Stroke 2000;31:601–9.

26. Abciximab Emergency Stroke Treatment Trial (AbESTT) Investigators. Emergency administration of abciximab for treatment of patients with acute ischemic stroke: results of a randomized phase 2 trial. Stroke 2005;36:880–90.

27. Adams HP Jr, Effron MB, Torner J, et al. Emergency administration of abciximab for treatment of patients with acute ischemic stroke: results of an international phase III trial: abciximab in Emergency Treatment of Stroke Trial (AbESTT-II). Stroke 2008;39:87–99.

28. Adams HP Jr, Leira EC, Torner JC, et al. Treating patients with "wake-up" stroke: the experience of the AbESTT-II trial. Stroke 2008;39:3277–82.

29. Siebler M, Hennerici MG, Schneider D, et al. Safety of Tirofiban in acute Ischemic Stroke: the SaTIS trial. Stroke 2011;42:2388–92.

30. Pancioli AM, Broderick J, Brott T, et al. The combined approach to lysis utilizing eptifibatide and rt-PA in acute ischemic stroke: the CLEAR stroke trial. Stroke 2008;39:3268–76.

31. Adams H, Adams R, Del Zoppo G, et al, Stroke Council of the American Heart Association, American Stroke Association. Guidelines for the early management of patients with ischemic stroke: 2005 guidelines update: a scientific statement from the Stroke Council of the American Heart Association/American Stroke Association. Stroke 2005;36:916–23.

32. Adams HP Jr, Adams RJ, Brott T, et al. Guidelines for the early management of patients with ischemic stroke: a scientific statement from the Stroke Council of the American Stroke Association. Stroke 2003;34:1056–83.

33. Adams HP Jr, Brott TG, Crowell RM, et al. Guidelines for the management of patients with acute ischemic stroke: a statement for healthcare professionals from a special writing group of the Stroke Council, American Heart Association. Circulation 1994;90:1588–601.

34. The European Stroke Organisation (ESO) Executive Committee, the ESO Writing Committee. Guidelines for management of ischaemic stroke and transient ischaemic attack 2008. Cerebrovasc Dis 2008;25:457–507.

35. Coull BM, Williams LS, Goldstein LB, et al. Anticoagulants and antiplatelet agents in acute ischemic stroke: report of the Joint Stroke Guideline Development Committee of the American Academy of Neurology and the American Stroke Association (a division of the American Heart Association). Neurology 2002;59:13–22.

36. Albers GW, Amarenco P, Easton JD, et al, American College of Chest Physicians. Antithrombotic and thrombolytic therapy for ischemic stroke: American College of Chest Physicians evidence-based clinical practice guidelines (8th edition). Chest 2008;133(Suppl):630S–69S.

37. EAFT (European Atrial Fibrillation Trial) Study Group. Secondary prevention in nonrheumatic atrial fibrillation after TIA or minor stroke. Lancet 1993;342:255–62.

38. Robert G, Hart MD, Santiago Palacio MD, et al. Atrial fibrillation, stroke, and acute antithrombotic therapy analysis of randomized clinical trials. Stroke 2002;33:2722–7.

39. Potter JF, Robinson TG, Ford GA, et al. Controlling hypertension and hypotension immediately poststroke (CHHIPS): a randomised, placebo-controlled, double-blind pilot trial. Lancet Neurol 2009;8:48–56.

40. Kaste M, Fogelholm R, Erilä T, et al. A randomized, double-blind, placebo-controlled trial of nimodipine in acute ischemic hemispheric stroke. Stroke 1994;25:1348–53.

41. Schrader J, Lüders S, Kulschewski A, et al, Acute Candesartan Cilexetil Therapy in Stroke Survivors Study Group. The ACCESS Study: evaluation of Acute Candesartan Cilexetil Therapy in Stroke Survivors. Stroke 2003;34:1699–703.

42. Robinson TG, Potter JF, Ford GA, et al, COSSACS Investigators. Effects of antihypertensive treatment after acute stroke in the Continue or Stop Post-Stroke Antihypertensives Collaborative Study (COSSACS): a prospective, randomised, open, blinded-endpoint trial. Lancet Neurol 2010;9:767–75.

43. He J, Zhang Y, Xu T, et al. Effects of immediate blood pressure reduction on death and major disability in patients with acute ischemic stroke: the CATIS randomized clinical trial. JAMA 2014;311:479–89.

44. Castillo J, Leira R, García MM, et al. Blood pressure decrease during the acute phase of ischemic stroke is associated with brain injury and poor stroke outcome. Stroke 2004;35:520–6.

45. Leonardi-Bee J, Bath PM, Phillips SJ, et al, IST Collaborative Group. Blood pressure and clinical outcomes in the International Stroke Trial. Stroke 2002;33:1315–20.

46. Okumura K, Ohya Y, Maehara A, et al. Effects of blood pressure levels on case fatality after acute stroke. J Hypertens 2005;23:1217–23.
47. Ginsberg MD, Palesch YY, Hill MD, et al. High-dose albumin treatment for acute ischaemic stroke (ALIAS) Part 2: a randomised, double-blind, phase 3, placebo-controlled trial. Lancet Neurol 2013;12:1049–58.
48. Shuaib A, Bornstein NM, Diener HC, et al, SENTIS Trial Investigators. Partial aortic occlusion for cerebral perfusion augmentation: safety and efficacy of NeuroFlo in Acute Ischemic Stroke trial. Stroke 2011;42:1680–90.
49. Han JH, Leung TW, Lam WW, et al. Preliminary findings of external counterpulsation for ischemic stroke patient with large artery occlusive disease. Stroke 2008;39:1340–3.
50. Rordorf G, Koroshetz WJ, Ezzeddine MA, et al. A pilot study of drug-induced hypertension for treatment of acute stroke. Neurology 2001;56:1210–3.
51. Marzan AS, Hungerbühler HJ, Studer A, et al. Feasibility and safety of norepinephrine-induced arterial hypertension in acute ischemic stroke. Neurology 2004;62:1193–5.
52. Shah QA, Patel S, Qureshi AI. Induced hypertension in patients with partial recanalization after intra-arterial thrombolysis for acute ischemic stroke. J Neurosurg Anesthesiol 2008;20:154–5.
53. Sherman DG. Prevention of venous thromboembolism, recurrent stroke and other vascular events after acute ischemic stroke: the role of low molecular weight heparin and antiplatelet therapy. J Stroke Cerebrovasc Dis 2006;15:250–9.
54. Sandercock PA, Counsell C, Tseng MC. Low molecular weight heparins or heparinoids versus standard unfractionated heparin for acute ischemic stroke. Cochrane Database Syst Rev 2008;(3):CD000119.
55. Shorr AF, Jackson WL, Sherner JH, et al. Differences between low molecular weight and unfractionated heparin for venous thromboembolism prevention following ischemic stroke: a metaanalysis. Chest 2008;133:149–55.
56. Andre C, De Freitas GR, Fukujima MM. Prevention of deep venous thrombosis and pulmonary embolism following stroke: a systematic review of published articles. Eur J Neurol 2007;14:21–32.
57. Azzimondi G, Bassein L, Nonino F, et al. Fever in acute stroke worsens prognosis: a prospective study. Stroke 1995;26:2040–3.
58. Castillo J, Dávalos A, Marrugat J, et al. Timing for fever-related brain damage in acute ischemic stroke. Stroke 1998;29:2455–60.
59. Prasad K, Krishnan PR. Fever is associated with doubling of odds of short-term mortality in ischemic stroke: an updated meta-analysis. Acta Neurol Scand 2010;122:404–8.
60. Diringer MN, Neurocritical Care Fever Reduction Trial Group. Treatment of fever in the neurologic intensive care unit with a catheter-based heat exchange system. Crit Care Med 2004;32:559–64.
61. Cryer PE, Davis SN, Shamoon H. Hypoglycemia in diabetes. Diabetes Care 2003;26:1902–12.
62. Service FJ. Hypoglycemic disorders. N Engl J Med 1995;332:1144–52.
63. Gray CS, Hildreth AJ, Sandercock PA, et al, GIST Trialists Collaboration. Glucose-potassium-insulin infusions in the management of post-stroke hyperglycaemia: the UK Glucose Insulin in Stroke Trial (GIST-UK). Lancet Neurol 2007;6:397–406.
64. American Diabetes Association. Standards of medical care in diabetes: 2010 [Erratum appears in Diabetes Care 2010;33:692]. Diabetes Care 2010;33(Suppl 1):S11–61.

65. Davenport RJ, Dennis MS, Warlow CP. Gastrointestinal hemorrhage after acute stroke. Stroke 1996;27:421–4.
66. Fadul CE, Lemann W, Thaler HT, et al. Perforation of the gastrointestinal tract in patients receiving steroids for neurological disease. Neurology 1988;38:348–52.
67. Inayet N, Amoateng-Adjepong Y, Upadya A, et al. Risks for developing critical illness with GI hemorrhage. Chest 2000;118:473–8.
68. Lu WY, Rhoney DH, Boling WB, et al. A review of stress ulcer prophylaxis in the neurosurgical intensive care unit. Neurosurgery 1997;41:416–25.
69. Tryba M, Cook D. Current guidelines on stress ulcer prophylaxis. Drugs 1997; 54:581–96.
70. Sulter G, Elting JW, Langedijk M, et al. Admitting acute ischemic stroke patients to a stroke care monitoring unit versus a conventional stroke unit: a randomized pilot study. Stroke 2003;34:101–4.
71. Cavallini A, Micieli G, Marcheselli S, et al. Role of monitoring in management of acute ischemic stroke patients. Stroke 2003;34:2599–603.
72. Christensen H, Fogh Christensen A, Boysen G. Abnormalities on ECG and telemetry predict stroke outcome at 3 months. J Neurol Sci 2005;234:99–103.
73. Lazzaro MA, Krishnan K, Prabhakaran S. Detection of atrial fibrillation with concurrent Holter monitoring and continuous cardiac telemetry following ischemic stroke and transient ischemic attack. J Stroke Cerebrovasc Dis 2012;21:89–93.
74. Kernan WN, Ovbiagele B, Black HR, et al. Guidelines for the prevention of stroke in patients with stroke and transient ischemic attack. Stroke 2014;45:2160–236.
75. Silvestrelli G, Parnetti L, Caso V, et al. Early admission to stroke unit influences clinical outcome. Eur J Neurol 2006;13:250–5.
76. Langhorne P, Pollock A. What are the components of effective stroke unit care? Age Ageing 2002;31:365–71.
77. Cadilhac DA, Ibrahim J, Pearce DC, et al, SCOPES Study Group. Multicenter comparison of processes of care between stroke units and conventional care wards in Australia. Stroke 2004;35:1035–40.
78. Bershad EM, Feen ES, Hernandez OH, et al. Impact of a specialized neurointensive care team on outcomes of critically ill acute ischemic stroke patients. Neurocrit Care 2008;9:287–92.
79. Gujjar AR, Deibert E, Manno EM, et al. Mechanical ventilation for ischemic stroke and intracerebral hemorrhage: indications, timing, and outcome. Neurology 1998;51:447–51.
80. Grotta J, Pasteur W, Khwaja G, et al. Elective intubation for neurologic deterioration after stroke. Neurology 1995;45:640–4.
81. Berrouschot J, Rossler A, Koster J, et al. Mechanical ventilation in patients with hemispheric stroke. Crit Care Med 2000;28:2956–61.
82. Milhaud D, Popp J, Thouvenot E, et al. Mechanical ventilation in ischemic stroke. J Stroke Cerebrovasc Dis 2004;13:183–8.
83. Kuzac N, Harrison DW, Zed PJ. Use of lidocaine and fentanyl premedication for neuroprotective rapid sequence intubation in the emergency department. CJEM 2006;8:80–4.
84. Clancy M, Halford S, Walls R, et al. In patients with head injuries who undergo rapid sequence intubation using succinylcholine, does pretreatment with a competitive neuromuscular blocking agent improve outcome? A literature review. Emerg Med J 2001;18:373–5.
85. Albanese J, Viviand X, Potie F, et al. Sulfentanil, fentanyl, and alfentanil in head trauma patients: a study on cerebral hemodynamics. Crit Care Med 1999;27: 407–11.

86. Stollings JL, Diedrich DA, Oyen LJ, et al. Rapid-sequence intubation: a review of the process and considerations when choosing medications. Ann Pharmacother 2014;48:62–76.
87. Priebe HJ. Use of cricoid pressure during rapid sequence induction: facts and fiction. Trends Anaesth Crit Care 2012;2:123–7.
88. The Acute Respiratory Distress Syndrome Network. Ventilation with lower tidal volumes as compared with traditional tidal volumes for acute lung injury and the acute respiratory distress syndrome. N Engl J Med 2000;342:1301–8.
89. Dellinger RP, Levy MM, Rhodes A, et al. Surviving Sepsis Campaign: international guidelines for management of severe sepsis and septic shock, 2012. Crit Care Med 2013;41:580–637.
90. Frank JI. Large hemispheric infarction, deterioration, and intracranial pressure. Neurology 1995;45:1286–90.
91. Hornig CR, Rust DS, Busse O, et al. Space-occupying cerebellar infarction: clinical course and prognosis. Stroke 1994;25:372–4.
92. Hacke W, Schwab S, Horn M. "Malignant" middle cerebral artery territory infarction: clinical course and prognostic signs. Arch Neurol 1996;53:309–15.
93. Huttner HB, Schwab S. Malignant middle cerebral infarction: clinical characteristics, treatment strategies, and future perspectives. Lancet Neurol 2009;8: 949–58.
94. Amarenco P. The spectrum of cerebellar infarctions. Neurology 1991;41:973–9.
95. Burns JD, Green DM, Metivier K, et al. Intensive care management of acute ischemic stroke. Emerg Med Clin North Am 2012;30:713–44.
96. Koenig MA, Bryan M, Lewin JL, et al. Reversal of transtentorial herniation with hypertonic saline. Neurology 2008;70:1023–9.
97. Kamal H, Navi BB, Nakagawa K, et al. Hypertonic saline versus mannitol for the treatment of elevated intracranial pressure: a meta-analysis of randomized controlled trials. Crit Care Med 2011;39:554–9.
98. Burn J, Dennis M, Bamford J, et al. Epileptic seizures after a first stroke: the Oxfordshire Community Stroke Project. BMJ 1997;315:1582–7.
99. Alberti A, Paciaroni M, Caso V, et al. Early seizures in patients with acute stroke: frequency, predictive factors, and effect on clinical outcome. Vasc Health Risk Manag 2008;4:715–20.
100. Brophy GM, Bell R, Claassen J, et al. Guidelines for the evaluation and management of status epilepticus. Neurocrit Care 2012;17:3–23.
101. Fairhead JF, Mehta Z, Rothwell PM. Population-based study of delays in carotid imaging and surgery and the risk of recurrent stroke. Neurology 2005;65:371–5.
102. Johansson EP, Wester P. Delay from symptoms to carotid endarterectomy. J Intern Med 2008;263:404–11.
103. Rerkasem K, Rothwell PM. Systematic review of the operative risks of carotid endarterectomy for recently symptomatic stenosis in relation to the timing of surgery. Stroke 2009;40:e564–72.
104. Ballotta E, Meneghetti G, Da Giau G, et al. Carotid endarterectomy within 2 weeks of minor ischemic stroke: a prospective study. J Vasc Surg 2008;48: 595–600.
105. Huber R, Müller BT, Seitz RJ, et al. Carotid surgery in acute symptomatic patients. Eur J Vasc Endovasc Surg 2003;25:60–7.
106. Paty PS, Darling RC 3rd, Feustel PJ, et al. Early carotid endarterectomy after acute stroke. J Vasc Surg 2004;39:148–54.
107. Sundt TM, Sandok BA, Whisnant JP. Carotid endarterectomy: complications and preoperative assessment of risk. Mayo Clin Proc 1975;50:301–6.

108. Biller J, Adams HP Jr, Boarini D, et al. Intraluminal clot of the carotid artery: a clinical-angiographic correlation of nine patients and literature review. Surg Neurol 1986;25:467–77.
109. Heros RC. Carotid endarterectomy in patients with intraluminal thrombus. Stroke 1988;19:667–8.
110. Buchan A, Gates P, Pelz D, et al. Intraluminal thrombus in the cerebral circulation: implications for surgical management. Stroke 1988;19:681–7.
111. Vahedi K, Hofmeijer J, Juettler E, et al. Early decompressive surgery in malignant infarction of the middle cerebral artery: a pooled analysis of three randomised controlled trials. Lancet Neurol 2007;6:215–22.
112. Juttler E, Unterberg A, Woitzik J, et al. Hemicraniectomy in older patients with extensive middle-cerebral-artery strokes. N Engl J Med 2014;370:1091–100.
113. Jauss M, Krieger D, Hornig C, et al. Surgical and medical management of patients with massive cerebellar infarctions: results of the German-Austrian cerebellar infarction study. J Neurol 1997;246:257–64.
114. Pfefferkorn T, Eppinger U, Linn J, et al. Long-term outcome after suboccipital decompressive craniectomy for malignant cerebellar infarction. Stroke 2009;40:3045–50.
115. Bershad EM, Suarez JI. Prothrombin complex concentrates for oral anticoagulation therapy-related intracranial hemorrhage: a review of the literature. Neurocrit Care 2010;12:403–13.

Critical Care Management of Intracerebral Hemorrhage

Sheila Chan, MD[a], J. Claude Hemphill III, MD, MAS[b,c],*

KEYWORDS

- Anticoagulants/adverse effects • Antihypertensive agents/therapeutic use
- Blood coagulation disorders • Intracerebral hemorrhage
- Hypertensive/diagnosis/cause/therapy • Neurocritical care
- Neurosurgical procedures

KEY POINTS

- Acute care of patients with intracerebral hemorrhage should prioritize stabilization of airway, breathing, and circulation; making a quick diagnosis; triage to an appropriate hospital unit; and measures to reduce risk of hematoma expansion, secondary neurologic deterioration, and complications of prolonged neurologic dysfunction.
- Physicians caring for patients with ICH should anticipate the need for emergent blood pressure reduction, coagulopathy reversal, cerebral edema management, and surgical interventions including ventriculostomy and hematoma evacuation.
- Neurologic aspects of critical care management extend to ventilation, cardiac monitoring, early feeding, infection surveillance, fever and hyperglycemia management, and venous thromboembolism prophylaxis.
- Early outcome prediction models are limited by the influence of elective withdrawal of care, do-not-resuscitate orders, and evolving effectiveness of new treatments.

Disclosures: The authors have no relevant financial disclosures. Dr J.C. Hemphill has several unrelated financial disclosures: research support from NIH/NINDS grant U10 NS058931 and Cerebrotech; stock and stock options from Ornim; consulting and speaking honoraria from Besins and Edge Therapeutics.

[a] Neurocritical Care Program, Department of Neurology, University of California, San Francisco, 1001 Potrero Avenue, San Francisco, CA 94110, USA; [b] Neurocritical Care Program, Department of Neurology, Brain and Spinal Injury Center, San Francisco General Hospital, University of California, San Francisco, Building 1, Room 101, 1001 Potrero Avenue, San Francisco, CA 94110, USA; [c] Department of Neurological Surgery, University of California, San Francisco, 1001 Potrero Avenue, San Francisco, CA 94110, USA
* Corresponding author. Department of Neurology, San Francisco General Hospital, Building 1, Room 101, 1001 Potrero Avenue, San Francisco, CA 94110.
E-mail address: chemphill@sfgh.ucsf.edu

Crit Care Clin 30 (2014) 699–717
http://dx.doi.org/10.1016/j.ccc.2014.06.003
0749-0704/14/$ – see front matter © 2014 Elsevier Inc. All rights reserved.

INTRODUCTION

Primary, spontaneous intracerebral hemorrhage (ICH) confers significant early mortality and long-term morbidity worldwide. The overall incidence is estimated at 24.6 cases per 100,000 person years, with a case fatality rate approximately 40% at 1 month and 54% at 1 year, and only 12% to 39% of patients achieving long-term functional independence.[1] A meta-analysis of ICH outcomes between 1980 and 2008 showed no appreciable change in case fatality rate over that time period, although retrospective studies of large cohorts in the United Kingdom and United States have shown a significant decrease in early mortality since 2000.[2,3] Decreases in 30-day and in-hospital mortality are possibly related to the introduction of improved investigative, diagnostic, and management strategies including bedside neuromonitoring, as well as ascertainment of less severe cases that may previously have been misdiagnosed as ischemic stroke. Example guidelines for the diagnosis and management of spontaneous ICH include those from the American Heart Association (American Stroke Association) and the Neurocritical Care Society (part of the Emergency Neurological Life Support [ENLS] program).[4,5] This article briefly reviews the pathogenesis and diagnosis of ICH, then details the acute management of spontaneous ICH in the critical care setting based on existing evidence and these published guidelines.

PATHOGENESIS

Spontaneous ICH results from the bursting of small intracerebral arteries, most commonly because of increased susceptibility to rupture caused by chronic vasculopathy.[6] Long-standing high blood pressure commonly leads to lipohyalinosis of tiny perforating arteries serving the thalamus, basal ganglia, and pons, causing deep hemorrhages that often extend into the ventricles.[7-9] In contrast, cerebral amyloid angiopathy (CAA) typically involves cortical perforators, and is the leading cause of lobar hemorrhage in patients more than 70 years of age.[10] Genetic alleles associated with high blood pressure and cerebral amyloid correlate with higher ICH risk, larger hematoma volume, and poor outcome.[9,11,12] Other common risk factors for spontaneous ICH include older age, history of stroke, history of heavy alcohol use, and education attainment at less than a high school level.[8,9] **Table 1** lists various primary and secondary causes of ICH.[13]

Table 1	
Causes of nontraumatic intracerebral hemorrhage	
Primary ICH	**Secondary ICH**
Hypertension	Vascular malformations
CAA	Arteriovenous malformation
Sympathomimetic drugs of	Cavernous malformation
abuse	Saccular aneurysm
Cocaine	Mycotic aneurysm
Methamphetamine	Dural arteriovenous fistula
Coagulopathy	Moyamoya
	Ischemic stroke (hemorrhagic conversion)
	Cerebral venous sinus thrombosis (hemorrhagic conversion)
	Tumor (primary or metastatic)
	Cerebral vasculitis

Data from Elijovich L, Patel PV, Hemphill JC 3rd. Intracerebral hemorrhage. Semin Neurol 2008;28(5):657–67.

Medications contribute significantly to the risk of ICH, larger hematoma volume, and ICH mortality. Warfarin use was associated with approximately 6.6% of ICH cases in the United States from 2005 to 2008, and this association is expected to increase as the population ages and more patients are placed on anticoagulants for a variety of cardiovascular indications.[3] Supratherapeutic warfarin use as measured by high International Normalized Ratio (INR) correlates with case rate and poor outcome.[8,9,14–16] Newer oral anticoagulants with lower potential for unpredictable therapeutic levels may confer less risk than warfarin.[17] Daily low-dose antiplatelet use, including clopidogrel use, confers a small increase in ICH risk, even when combined with warfarin.[8,18] Although premorbid statin use has not been related to ICH outcome, low low-density lipoprotein is associated with in-hospital mortality, and high-dose atorvastatin may be associated with recurrent ICH.[9,19,20]

ICH commonly occurs in the putamen (46%), followed by thalamic (18%), lobar (9%), caudate (4%), pontine (13%), cerebellar (4%), and primary ventricular (2%) locations.[21] Lobar hemorrhage has a predilection for the occipital lobes, followed by frontal, temporal, and parietal lobes.[10] Lobar hemorrhage is more often associated with recurrent ICH than deep hemorrhage.[16]

The initial neurologic damage to tissue at the epicenter of ICH formation is unlikely to be salvaged because of blood dissection causing direct and rapid tissue destruction. The first few days after acute ICH confer additional threat of neurologic worsening caused by hematoma expansion, edema, and resultant secondary brain injury. Secondary injury from inflammation, red cell lysis, and disruption of the blood-brain barrier can compromise the surrounding brain parenchyma.[22] Perihematoma edema develops early after ICH, can double within the first 7 to 11 days, and may persist for 4 weeks, even with small-volume ICH.[23,24] The degree of edema is associated with poor outcome.

DIAGNOSIS

The diagnosis of ICH is suspected on the sudden onset of acute focal neurologic symptoms. The constellation of findings typically relates to the location of the hematoma and its impact on the surrounding brain parenchyma, and is indistinguishable from acute ischemic stroke or other paroxysmal neurologic disorders without neuroimaging.[5] The clinical presentation of ICH may also include acute severe headache, vomiting, seizure, high systolic blood pressure (SBP) greater than 220 mm Hg, and rapid deterioration in consciousness, although none of these are specific for ICH.[4] A brief medical history should also include inquiry for anticoagulant use, recent head trauma, prior stroke, and other hemorrhage.

In addition to an expeditious clinical history and neurologic examination, a swift neuroimaging test is necessary to diagnosis primary ICH quickly and to initiate appropriate acute management. Time from symptom onset to scan is associated with long-term mortality.[18] A computed tomography (CT) study of the head performed without contrast is usually the most efficient study for diagnosis, and may provide further information helpful for clinical decision making. The presence of an intra-axial, hyperdense consolidated lesion is extremely sensitive (89%) and specific (100%) for acute ICH.[25] Hematoma volume is easily estimated using the ABC/2 method (A, maximum hematoma diameter of a reference axial slice that appears largest in hematoma area; B, maximum hematoma diameter perpendicular to A; and C, number of slices in vertical plane with hematoma multiplied by slice thickness [with slices <25% in hematoma volume of the reference slice being ignored, those 25% to 75% of the reference slice considered as a half slice, and those >75% considered a full slice]).

Although highly variable, the ABC/2 method is reliable for most clinical decision making.[26,27] Large hematoma volumes and the presence of heterogeneous ICH attenuation are predictive of subsequent hematoma expansion.[28,29] Gradient echo and T2* susceptibility magnetic resonance imaging (MRI) may be equivalent to CT in the diagnosis of acute ICH, although availability of MRI and the clinical condition of many acute patients with ICH often limit the use of MRI as the primary imaging modality (**Fig. 1**).

The addition of contrast to the head CT may show a spot sign, which represents active contrast extravasation into the hematoma and has a 60% association with hematoma expansion (**Fig. 2**).[30] The spot-and-tail sign, a linear density extending from the first segment of the middle cerebral artery into the hematoma and coursing toward the spot sign, may be even more sensitive for predicting hematoma expansion and acute deterioration.[31] CT angiogram/venogram performed with contrast during the acute phase has an overall sensitivity of 97.0% and specificity of 98.9% for causal vascular abnormalities, compared with digital subtraction angiography (DSA) as the gold standard.[32] Other CT findings, such as the presence of subarachnoid

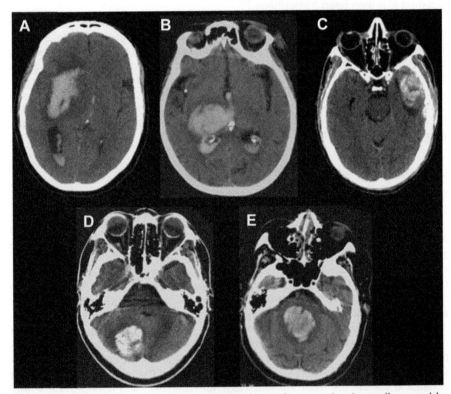

Fig. 1. Typical locations for ICH. ICH caused by chronic hypertension is usually caused by rupture of small penetrating arterioles and typically occurs in the basal ganglia (*A*), thalamus (*B*), cerebellum (*D*), and pons (*E*). ICH from CAA and sympathomimetic drugs of abuse such as cocaine or methamphetamine often occurs in lobar regions such as the temporal lobe (*C*). Supratentorial ICH is considered as basal ganglia, thalamic, or lobar (*A–C*), whereas ICH originating in the cerebellum or pons is considered infratentorial (*D* and *E*). Intraventricular hemorrhage (IVH) can also be seen (*A–C, E*). (*Reproduced from* Andrews CM, Jauch EC, Hemphill JC 3rd, et al. Emergency neurological life support: intracerebral hemorrhage. Neurocrit Care 2012;17 Suppl 1:S39; with permission.)

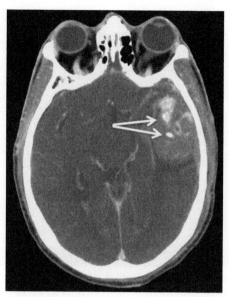

Fig. 2. Contrast extravasation (spot sign) in acute ICH. In this postcontrast image obtained after administration of intravenous contrast during a stroke CT scan (noncontrast study, CT angiogram, CT perfusion study), contrast extravasation is present in this acute left temporal lobe ICH. This feature is commonly referred to as a spot sign (*arrows*) and is associated with increased risk of hematoma expansion. (*Reproduced from* Andrews CM, Jauch EC, Hemphill JC 3rd, et al. Emergency neurological life support: intracerebral hemorrhage. Neurocrit Care 2012;17 Suppl 1:S40; with permission.)

hemorrhage, subdural hemorrhage, intraventricular hemorrhage (IVH), and leukoaraiosis are associated with early and long-term mortality.[16,33,34]

MRI performed in the subacute stage of the disease is highly accurate for detecting underlying vascular malformations, and also provides valuable information regarding other causes of intracerebral hemorrhage such as CAA, cavernoma, arterial hypertension, hemorrhagic transformation of ischemic infarct, and malignant brain tumor.[35] The presence of microbleeds on MRI is associated with increased risk of hematoma expansion, likely from vasculopathy caused by amyloid angiopathy or chronic hypertension (**Fig. 3**).[36] Magnetic resonance (MR) angiography is nearly equivalent to DSA for diagnosing vascular abnormalities.[37] Patients 55 years of age or less, without a history of hypertension, or with lobar hemorrhage should routinely undergo MRI/MR angiography.[37] Repeat studies at a later date are recommended if there is concern that an underlying lesion cannot be ruled out because of the presence of unresorbed blood. There is no consensus on the ideal timing for MRI, but lesions have been found on imaging performed earlier than 20 days and longer than 100 days from the acute hemorrhage. DSA is considered the gold standard for vascular abnormalities, and should be performed if the clinical suspicion is high and the screening MR or CT is suggestive.

The initial evaluation should also include laboratory studies of coagulopathy, blood count, and toxicology screen to identify additional contributors to ICH, and to assess the need for reversal. Careful review of the clinical history, physical examination, neuroimaging, and laboratory studies may reveal more rare causes of ICH including angiitis, autonomic dysreflexia, connective tissue disease, infection with bacteremia and endocarditis, and moyamoya disease.[38–42]

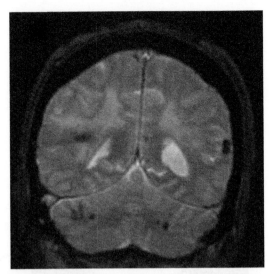

Fig. 3. Cerebral microhemorrhages in a patient with CAA. MRI T2 susceptibility-weighted images showing several asymptomatic microhemorrhages scattered throughout the cerebral and cerebellar hemispheres. (*Reproduced from* Elijovich L, Patel PV, Hemphill JC 3rd. Intra-cerebral hemorrhage. Semin Neurol 2008;28(5):661; with permission.)

ACUTE MANAGEMENT

The severe acuity of suspected ICH often necessitates emergent medical assessment before a definitive diagnosis of ICH is made. Acute management protocols such as ENLS prioritize stabilization of airway, breathing, and circulation (ABCs), making a quick diagnosis, triage to an appropriate hospital unit, and measures to reduce risk of hematoma expansion, secondary neurologic deterioration, and complications of prolonged neurologic dysfunction. In addition, certain ICH-specific issues need to be addressed rapidly and these are emphasized in the ENLS checklist for ICH (**Box 1**).

ABCs

Patients who are obtunded or comatose may require immediate airway management before they are stable enough to undergo neuroimaging. Rapid sequence intubation should be undertaken for patients who cannot protect their airway because of poor

---

Box 1
ENLS ICH checklist for the first hour after diagnosis

- Blood pressure
- PT, PTT, platelet count, INR
- Head CT: measure size of hemorrhage (ABC/2 method)
- Calculate Glasgow Coma Scale score
- Determine ICH score

Abbreviations: PT, prothrombin time; PTT, partial thromboplastin time.
   Data from Andrews CM, Jauch EC, Hemphill JC 3rd, et al. Emergency neurological life support: intracerebral hemorrhage. Neurocrit Care 2012;17 Suppl 1:S37–46.

mental status, impaired gag and swallow reflexes, or severe vomiting. Barring any significant pulmonary disease, intubated patients can be managed with minimal mechanical ventilator support.

Blood Pressure

Prospective studies show that extreme increases in blood pressure in the immediate time period after ICH predict hematoma expansion and early neurologic deterioration.[43,44] The results of the Intensive Blood Pressure Reduction in Acute Cerebral Hemorrhage Trial 2 (INTERACT2) showed that patients randomized to early intensive lowering of blood pressure to target SBP less than 140 mm Hg (compared with a target SBP of 180 mm Hg) had no difference in death or major disability at 90 days, but significantly better 90-day modified Rankin scores.[45] Aggressive blood pressure management strategies have not been shown to reduce hematoma volumes or perihematoma cerebral blood flow.[46] Nevertheless, early aggressive blood pressure management strategies seem to be safe, and targets of SBP less than 140 mm Hg are reasonable to maximize patient outcomes.[47] Commonly used medications include intravenous β-blockers and calcium channel blockers. Nitrates should be avoided because of potential for cerebral vasodilation, impaired cerebral autoregulation and increased intracranial pressure (ICP). Close blood pressure monitoring and frequent medication titrations are necessary to avoid overshoot and to ensure that cerebral perfusion pressure is maintained in cases of increased ICP.[5] A blood pressure control protocol initiated in the emergency department with early arterial line placement, continued in an intensive care unit, is encouraged to safely and rapidly achieve target blood pressure parameters.[48]

Coagulopathy

Although coagulopathy is associated with worse outcomes, acute reversal of coagulopathy has not been clearly shown to result in clinical benefit. Even though this area has not been extensively studied in large randomized trials, existing guidelines emphasize rapid correction of coagulopathy in potentially salvageable patients. Options for correction of an INR greater than 1.4 caused by warfarin include fresh-frozen plasma (FFP), vitamin K, prothrombin complex concentrates (PCC), or recombinant activated factor 7 (rFVIIa). Vitamin K is administered slowly in doses of 5 to 10 mg intravenously. It has long-lasting effects and should be given to all eligible patients; however, it is insufficient for rapid INR correction. Monitoring for a severe anaphylactic reaction during infusion is essential. PCCs can be administered more quickly than FFP, correct the INR faster, and require less volume of infusion.[49] Recombinant factor VIIa is not recommended as a singular agent for warfarin reversal because this may correct the INR value, but not completely correct the coagulopathy. In addition, the Factor Seven for Acute Hemorrhagic Stroke Trial (FAST) in patients with noncoagulopathic ICH showed that rFVIIa in doses of 20 and 80 μg/kg resulted in significant reduction in hematoma expansion at 24 hours, but no significant difference in rate of poor clinical outcome. Although serious thromboembolic events were the same in all treatment groups, arterial events were more frequent in those receiving 80 μg/kg of rFVIIa versus placebo.[50] Thus, the use of rFVIIa is not routinely recommended for any category of patients with ICH.

Optimal coagulopathy reversal of newer oral anticoagulants remains unclarified. The effect of dabigatran might be partially reversed by PCC, rFVIIa, activated charcoal, and hemodialysis. Rivaroxaban and apixaban are more likely to be partially reversed by PCC.[51] Practitioners should also be aware of the type of PCC available in their facilities. PCC may include 3 factors (II, IX, and X) or 4 factors (II, VII, IX, and

X); some 4-factor PCCs include small amounts of heparin and should be avoided in patients with heparin-induced thrombocytopenia. Although patients on clopidogrel, and possibly aspirin, may be at risk for increased hematoma volumes and higher in-hospital mortality, the clinical benefit of platelet transfusions or 1-deamino-8-D-arginine vasopressin (DDAVP), either empirically or targeted using platelet function assays, have not been clearly shown in the limited studies to date.[52,53]

Neurocritical Care

Retrospective reviews show that more than 20% of patients with ICH deteriorate within the first 2 days of presentation.[54,55] Patients with large hematoma volume, IVH, midline shift on head CT, high blood pressure requiring frequent administrations of medications and close blood pressure monitoring, hyperglycemia, and alterations in consciousness are at higher risk of hematoma expansion and neurologic worsening, and should be considered for immediate transfer to a multidisciplinary neurocritical care unit or tertiary care center, if available. Physicians caring for patients with ICH/IVH might anticipate the need for surgical interventions such as ventriculostomy and hematoma evacuation, which are often prompted by findings on repeat neurologic examination in the acute period after hemorrhage.[56] Although the evidence on unimodality and multimodality neuromonitoring in ICH is limited, management targets derived from traumatic brain injury research may aid with prevention, early detection, and treatment of secondary brain injury.[57] Neurocritical care services have been shown to more effectively perform blood pressure management and dysphagia screening, and may be associated with improved in-hospital mortality.[58,59] Stabilization of ABCs, initiation of blood pressure management, and measures to reverse coagulopathy should be initiated before transfer to a higher level of care. Close communication on the clinical status of the patient and plans for care are paramount to effective transfer either within a hospital or to another hospital.

Repeat Imaging

A prospective study of repeat imaging showed that delayed IVH occurred in 21% of patients with ICH without initial IVH, and that these patients did as poorly as those with initial IVH. Furthermore, delayed findings occurred up to 72 hours from the time of symptom onset.[60] A protocol for repeat imaging is recommended in anticipation of the need for emergent procedures such as ventriculostomy and management of hydrocephalus and increased ICP. The optimal timing and number of repeat studies is unclear, and should be guided by close monitoring of neurologic signs.

Ventriculostomy and ICP Management

Hydrocephalus complicates up to 50% of ICH cases, and is associated with younger age, lower Glasgow Coma Scale score, deep hemorrhages, intubation, and mortality.[61] Patients with ICH with a Glasgow Coma Scale (GCS) score less than 9, those with clinical evidence of transtentorial herniation, or those with significant IVH or hydrocephalus may be considered for ventriculostomy to monitor ICP, titrate ICP treatment, and drain intraventricular blood.[4] In a retrospective review, ICP greater than 20 mm Hg occurred in 70% of patients with ICH who had an ICP monitor placed, and was most common in young patients with supratentorial hemorrhage.[62] ICP variability with active treatment is associated with poor outcome at 30 days and inpatient mortality, but not 12-month outcome.[63] Increased ICP may be treated with hyperosmolar therapy such as intravenous hypertonic saline or mannitol, cerebrospinal fluid drainage, or sedation, although none of these have been shown to improve functional outcome.[64,65] A retrospective review of 64 patients with ICH who received intraventricular recombinant tissue plasminogen activator (rT-PA) in doses of 8 ± 6 mg showed safety, although in-hospital mortality and cerebral edema was unchanged compared with matched controls.[66] The High Dose Deferoxamine in ICH (HI-DEF) trial is underway to follow up a phase I trial that showed that deferoxamine mesylate dosed at 62 mg/kg/d may exert neuroprotective effects, reduce perihematoma edema and neuronal damage, and improve functional recovery without increase in serious adverse event or mortality.[67]

Surgical Interventions

Certain patients with ICH may benefit from surgical evacuation of the hematoma, although prospective randomized trials in patients with supratentorial ICH have not shown significant benefit in the patients studied. The International Surgical Trial in Intracerebral Haemorrhage (STICH) did not show benefit on mortality or 6-month functional outcome of a policy of early hematoma evacuation of supratentorial ICH.[68] STICH II studied early hematoma evacuation in a subset of patients with lobar ICH, hematoma volumes 10 to 100 mL, and without IVH. The trial showed no overall significant difference in combined death or disability compared with initial conservative treatment, although a subgroup of patients with an initial poor prognosis may have benefitted.[69]

Because of high morbidity, cerebellar hemorrhages in patients with neurologic deterioration should be evacuated and this is recommended per current guidelines.[4,5] Preoperative risk stratification using the ICH Score may predict surgical outcome and assist with patient selection.[70] If surgery is indicated, INR should generally be corrected to less than 1.5 and platelet count to greater than 100,000 per microliter with transfusions as needed.[71]

Other surgical procedures may be helpful in reducing hematoma volume, ICP, and midline shift. Small case series have shown the feasibility of decompressive hemicraniectomy, with or without clot evacuation.[72–74] The transsylvian-transinsular approach is a minimally invasive method that can visualize a bleeding vessel under the microscope, spare functional cortex, and achieve high hematoma clearance rate with adequate decompression.[75] Image-guided needle-based approaches with robot control also debulk hematoma while sparing healthy brain tissue.[76] The ongoing Minimally Invasive Surgery Plus rt-PA for Intracerebral Hemorrhage Evacuation (MISTIE) trial combines stereotactic catheter placement and clot aspiration with injections of rt-PA through the catheter every 8 hours, up to 9 doses or until clot reduction end point. The procedure seems to be safe and the trial is ongoing as of this writing.[77]

Seizure Monitoring and Anticonvulsant Treatment

Retrospective reviews report electrographic seizures in up to one-third of patients monitored with continuous electroencephalography (EEG), with about half of seizures being electrographic only and most occurring within the first 24 hours after ICH. Seizures are associated with younger age, hemicraniectomy, ventriculostomy, intubation, tracheostomy, lower in-hospital mortality, and longer hospital length of stay.[78,79] Evidence is unclear about the effect of seizures on overall outcomes; whether seizures should be treated; and, if so, with which anticonvulsant medications. Retrospective data about anticonvulsant treatment are confounded by indication, disease severity, and do-not-resuscitate (DNR) status.[80] A prospective review of patients given anticonvulsants showed that phenytoin was associated with more fever and worse outcomes.[81] EEG monitoring is probably indicated in patients with ICH with depressed mental status out of proportion to the degree of brain injury. Patients with clinically significant seizures should be treated with anticonvulsants, but prophylactic medications, especially phenytoin, are not generally recommended.[4]

Cardiac Monitoring

Patients with ICH should receive close cardiac monitoring for the first few days, especially if they are undergoing active management for blood pressure using intravenous medications. In a retrospective review, most electrocardiographic changes occurred in patients with ICH with deep hemorrhage. QTc and ST abnormalities, and bradyarrhythmias/tachyarrhythmias were common. Almost all patients with IVH had QTc prolongation and this has been associated with in-hospital mortality regardless of IVH. ST segment abnormalities were also associated with higher in-hospital mortality.[82] Wall motion abnormalities in patients with ICH are frequently seen on transthoracic echocardiogram. They are associated with lower admission SBP, history of ischemic heart disease, but not in-hospital mortality, age, gender, GCS, or hematoma volume. Routine transthoracic echocardiography is unlikely to be helpful for treatment course, but may be helpful in cases of high clinical suspicion or a history of ischemic heart disease.[83]

Mechanical Ventilation

In retrospective reviews, up to 21% of patients with ICH are mechanically ventilated, usually for inability to protect the airway because of poor level of consciousness. Intubated patients with ICH are at risk for pulmonary edema, acute respiratory distress syndrome (ARDS), pneumonia, and long-term need for tracheostomy.[84] Ventilated patients have as much as 48% in-hospital mortality, and death rates after discharge are high. However, up to 42% of ventilated patients who survive to discharge have a good functional outcome.[85]

ARDS has a prevalence of about 27% in intubated patients with ICH and usually occurs by hospital day 2, with a pathophysiology possibly related to neurogenic pulmonary edema. ARDS in patients with ICH is associated with high tidal volumes, male sex, blood transfusions, higher fluid balance, obesity, hypoxemia, acidosis, tobacco use, emergent hematoma evacuation, and vasopressor dependence. Lower GCS is not associated, suggesting that aspiration is not a significant contributor. ARDS is also not independently associated with in-hospital mortality or functional outcome, possibly because the morbidity of ICH is already so high.[86,87] Management of ARDS in patients with ICH must balance the risks of hypercapnea with hypoxia as related to secondary brain injury.

Intubated patients should undergo surveillance for ventilator-associated pneumonia along with pneumonia-prevention measures such as minimizing duration of mechanical ventilation, health care personnel hand hygiene, head of bed elevation to 30°, and good oral care.[88] Patients progressing to tracheostomy tend to have larger hematoma volumes, IVH, hydrocephalus, low admission GCS, pneumonia, and intubation period longer than 2 weeks. Prediction models for timing of tracheostomy have the potential to reduce complications of endotracheal intubation and decrease hospital length of stay.

Nutrition

In a retrospective review of patients with ICH divided into enteral feeding initiated within 48 hours versus delayed feeding, in-hospital mortality was lower in the early feeding group, as were pneumonia, sepsis, discharge morbidity, and intensive care unit length of stay.[89] Efforts should be undertaken to feed patients with ICH as early as safely possible.

Hyperglycemia, Hypothermia

Blood glucose greater than 140 mg/dL and temperature greater than 37.5°C at hospital admission predict late neurologic deterioration.[54,55] Although aggressive treatment of these parameters has not been systematically investigated for ICH, maintenance of normothermia and euglycemia are reasonable strategies for minimizing secondary brain injury.

Infection

Infection in patients with ICH is associated with worse clinical status, larger hematoma volumes, IVH, and invasive procedures. Common infections include pneumonia, urinary tract infection, and clinical or laboratory evidence of infection without identified source.[90] Patients should undergo active monitoring for infections with aggressive treatment when indicated by clinical status.

Venous Thromboembolism Prophylaxis

The incidence of symptomatic venous thromboembolism ranges from 0.5% to 13% of patients with ICH, and pulmonary embolism from 0.7% to 5%. Hemiplegic patients may have rates of asymptomatic thromboembolism as high as 75%. In a pilot study, 97 patients with ICH received low-molecular-weight heparin by 36 hours of admission as long as they were free of clinical or radiological growth of hemorrhage. None developed fatal embolism, 2 patients had moderate hematoma growth, and 2 developed nonsignificant heparin-induced thrombocytopenia.[91] Early venous thromboembolism prophylaxis with intermittent pneumatic compression devices, elastic stockings, and low-molecular-weight heparin or unfractionated heparin is probably reasonable and safe for immobile patients.

Blood Transfusion

Anemia has a 25% prevalence in patients with ICH, which is much higher than in the general elderly population, and is correlated with poor functional outcome.[92] It is not clear whether transfusions are helpful.[93]

Outcome Predictions

Despite improvements in acute care, ICH continues to be a disease with high morbidity and mortality. Outcome prediction models seek to accurately identify patients who might survive and benefit from acute and long-term care. The ICH Score, ICH Grading Scale, and Modified ICH Score have all been evaluated in multiple retrospective cohorts and are highly predictive of 30-day mortality (**Table 2**).[94–96] However, the point estimates from the original publications of all of these are limited by the influence of elective withdrawal of support and DNR orders.[97,98] Even so, the use of a baseline severity score such as one of these or the FUNC score is reasonable because this may help with communication across caregivers and with patient families.[99] Patients who progress to brain death may be eligible for organ donation, and loss of brainstem reflexes or the CT swirl sign on admission may aid in early identification.[100] Longer term functional outcome has also been correlated with neuroimaging cerebral volume loss, transcranial Doppler pulsatility index, hematoma involvement of the inferior parietal lobule or posterior insula, surgical feeding tube placement, and tracheostomy placement, but none of these are individually sensitive or specific.[101–104]

In a prospective registry of 245 patients, 18% had DNR orders instituted within 24 hours of admission. DNR cases did not receive ventricular drainage or surgical hematoma evacuation. By matched analysis, more controls had surgical evacuation and

Table 2 Determination of the ICH score	
Component	ICH Score Points
GCS	
3–4	2
5–12	1
13–15	0
ICH Volume (mL)	
≥30	1
<30	0
Intraventricular Hemorrhage	
Yes	1
No	0
Infratentorial Origin of ICH	
Yes	1
No	0
Age (y)	
≥80	1
<80	0
Total ICH score	0–6

Data from Hemphill JC 3rd, Bonovich DC, Besmertis L, et al. The ICH score: a simple, reliable grading scale for intracerebral hemorrhage. Stroke 2001;32(4):891–7.

mechanical ventilation, but there was no difference in functional outcome and survival at 1 year.[105] Current guidelines recommend aggressive full care and avoiding new DNR orders until at least the second day of hospitalization in order to decrease the likelihood of a self-fulfilling prophecy of poor outcome caused by early care limitations.[4]

LONG-TERM MANAGEMENT

Patients who survive to discharge should receive aggressive rehabilitation as tolerated to maximize functional outcome. Long-term management of identified risk factors such as hypertension, alcohol use, and other substance abuse are important to reduce ICH recurrence risk.

For patients who were on anticoagulation or antiplatelet therapy at the time of hemorrhage, the evidence on restarting therapy is limited. Retrospective studies show no differences in strokes among patients who did or did not resume anticoagulation.[106] For patients with lobar hemorrhage and nonvalvular atrial fibrillation, avoidance of long-term anticoagulation is reasonable because of the high risk of ICH recurrence, especially in the setting of CAA.[4] Newer anticoagulants may have advantages but lack effective laboratory testing and availability of reversal agents.[107] Each patient must be assessed individually according to the underlying medical condition, hemorrhagic burden, comorbidities, and complication risks.

Regarding statins, secondary analysis of the Stroke Prevention by Aggressive Reduction in Cholesterol Levels (SPARCL) trial suggested that statins were associated with occurrence of ICH primarily in patients with a history of ICH.[20] Nevertheless, the overall benefit of stroke risk reduction and coronary events with atorvastatin dosed at

80 mg/d likely outweighs the increase in ICH.[108] Another extensive meta-analysis found no association between statins and ICH occurrence.[109] Retrospective reviews show that patients exposed to statins as early as 72 hours after hemorrhage onset have reduced death and disability at 1 year, and those who receive low doses of atorvastatin at 20 mg/d have no increased risk of recurrent ICH.[110,111] Thus, it is probably safe to restart low-dose statin treatment early after ICH, and increase the dose as clinically appropriate.

SUMMARY

Despite the high morbidity and mortality of ICH, advances in acute management have contributed greatly to the improved survival potential of patients with ICH. High-quality care based on evidence and delivered by practitioners familiar with practice guidelines is paramount to maximizing functional outcomes. Acute ICH management will continue to evolve with ongoing research on ICH treatments and neurocritical care.

REFERENCES

1. van Asch CJ, Luitse MJ, Rinkel GJ, et al. Incidence, case fatality, and functional outcome of intracerebral haemorrhage over time, according to age, sex, and ethnic origin: a systematic review and meta-analysis. Lancet Neurol 2010;9(2): 167–76.
2. Gonzalez-Perez A, Gaist D, Wallander MA, et al. Mortality after hemorrhagic stroke: data from general practice (The Health Improvement Network). Neurology 2013;81(6):559–65.
3. Liotta EM, Prabhakaran S. Warfarin-associated intracerebral hemorrhage is increasing in prevalence in the United States. J Stroke Cerebrovasc Dis 2013; 22(7):1151–5.
4. Morgenstern LB, Hemphill JC 3rd, Anderson C, et al. Guidelines for the management of spontaneous intracerebral hemorrhage: a guideline for healthcare professionals from the American Heart Association/American Stroke Association. Stroke 2010;41(9):2108–29.
5. Andrews CM, Jauch EC, Hemphill JC 3rd, et al. Emergency neurological life support: intracerebral hemorrhage. Neurocrit Care 2012;17(Suppl 1):S37–46.
6. Fisher CM. Pathological observations in hypertensive cerebral hemorrhage. J Neuropathol Exp Neurol 1971;30(3):536–50.
7. Chiquete E, Ochoa-Guzman A, Vargas-Sanchez A, et al. Blood pressure at hospital admission and outcome after primary intracerebral hemorrhage. Arch Med Sci 2013;9(1):34–9.
8. Garcia-Rodriguez LA, Gaist D, Morton J, et al. Antithrombotic drugs and risk of hemorrhagic stroke in the general population. Neurology 2013;81(6):566–74.
9. Martini SR, Flaherty ML, Brown WM, et al. Risk factors for intracerebral hemorrhage differ according to hemorrhage location. Neurology 2012;79(23):2275–82.
10. Charidimou A, Gang Q, Werring DJ. Sporadic cerebral amyloid angiopathy revisited: recent insights into pathophysiology and clinical spectrum. J Neurol Neurosurg Psychiatr 2012;83(2):124–37.
11. Falcone GJ, Biffi A, Devan WJ, et al. Burden of blood pressure-related alleles is associated with larger hematoma volume and worse outcome in intracerebral hemorrhage. Stroke 2013;44(2):321–6.
12. Devan WJ, Falcone GJ, Anderson CD, et al. Heritability estimates identify a substantial genetic contribution to risk and outcome of intracerebral hemorrhage. Stroke 2013;44(6):1578–83.

13. Elijovich L, Patel PV, Hemphill JC 3rd. Intracerebral hemorrhage. Semin Neurol 2008;28(5):657–67.
14. Horstmann S, Rizos T, Lauseker M, et al. Intracerebral hemorrhage during anti-coagulation with vitamin K antagonists: a consecutive observational study. J Neurol 2013;260(8):2046–51.
15. Ma M, Meretoja A, Churilov L, et al. Warfarin-associated intracerebral hemorrhage: volume, anticoagulation intensity and location. J Neurol Sci 2013;332(1–2):75–9.
16. Tveiten A, Ljostad U, Mygland A, et al. Leukoaraiosis is associated with short- and long-term mortality in patients with intracerebral hemorrhage. J Stroke Cerebrovasc Dis 2013;22(7):919–25.
17. Chatterjee J, Sardar P, Biondi-Zoccai G, et al. New oral anticoagulants and the risk of intracranial hemorrhage: traditional and Bayesian meta-analysis and mixed treatment comparison of randomized trials of new oral anticoagulants in atrial fibrillation. JAMA Neurol 2013;70(12):1486–90.
18. Falcone GJ, Biffi A, Brouwers HB, et al. Predictors of hematoma volume in deep and lobar supratentorial intracerebral hemorrhage. JAMA Neurol 2013;70(8):988–94.
19. Mustanoja S, Strbian D, Putaala J, et al. Association of prestroke statin use and lipid levels with outcome of intracerebral hemorrhage. Stroke 2013;44(8):2330–2.
20. Goldstein LB, Amarenco P, Szarek M, et al. Hemorrhagic stroke in the Stroke Prevention by Aggressive Reduction in Cholesterol Levels study. Neurology 2008;70(24 Pt 2):2364–70.
21. Nah HW, Kwon SU, Kang DW, et al. Moyamoya disease-related versus primary intracerebral: hemorrhage location and outcomes are different. Stroke 2012;43(7):1947–50.
22. Ziai WC. Hematology and inflammatory signaling of intracerebral hemorrhage. Stroke 2013;44(6 Suppl 1):S74–8.
23. Qureshi AI, Majidi S, Gilani WI, et al. Increased brain volume among good grade patients with intracerebral hemorrhage. Results from the Antihypertensive Treatment of Acute Cerebral Hemorrhage (ATACH) Study. Neurocrit Care 2013;20(3):470–5.
24. Staykov D, Wagner I, Volbers B, et al. Natural course of perihemorrhagic edema after intracerebral hemorrhage. Stroke 2011;42(9):2625–9.
25. Chalela JA, Kidwell CS, Nentwich LM, et al. Magnetic resonance imaging and computed tomography in emergency assessment of patients with suspected acute stroke: a prospective comparison. Lancet 2007;369(9558):293–8.
26. Kothari RU, Brott T, Broderick JP, et al. The ABCs of measuring intracerebral hemorrhage volumes. Stroke 1996;27(8):1304–5.
27. Hussein HM, Tariq NA, Palesch YY, et al. Reliability of hematoma volume measurement at local sites in a multicenter acute intracerebral hemorrhage clinical trial. Stroke 2013;44(1):237–9.
28. Barras CD, Tress BM, Christensen S, et al. Quantitative CT densitometry for predicting intracerebral hemorrhage growth. AJNR Am J Neuroradiol 2013;34(6):1139–44.
29. Takeda R, Ogura T, Ooigawa H, et al. A practical prediction model for early hematoma expansion in spontaneous deep ganglionic intracerebral hemorrhage. Clin Neurol Neurosurg 2013;115(7):1028–31.
30. Rizos T, Dorner N, Jenetzky E, et al. Spot signs in intracerebral hemorrhage: useful for identifying patients at risk for hematoma enlargement? Cerebrovasc Dis 2013;35(6):582–9.

31. Sorimachi T, Osada T, Baba T, et al. The striate artery, hematoma, and spot sign on coronal images of computed tomography angiography in putaminal intracerebral hemorrhage. Stroke 2013;44(7):1830–2.

32. Wong GK, Siu DY, Abrigo JM, et al. Computed tomographic angiography for patients with acute spontaneous intracerebral hemorrhage. J Clin Neurosci 2012; 19(4):498–500.

33. Maas MB, Nemeth AJ, Rosenberg NF, et al. Subarachnoid extension of primary intracerebral hemorrhage is associated with poor outcomes. Stroke 2013;44(3): 653–7.

34. Kim BJ, Lee SH, Ryu WS, et al. Extents of white matter lesions and increased intraventricular extension of intracerebral hemorrhage. Crit Care Med 2013; 41(5):1325–31.

35. Lummel N, Lutz J, Bruckmann H, et al. The value of magnetic resonance imaging for the detection of the bleeding source in non-traumatic intracerebral haemorrhages: a comparison with conventional digital subtraction angiography. Neuroradiology 2012;54(7):673–80.

36. Marti-Fabregas J, Delgado-Mederos R, Granell E, et al. Microbleed burden and hematoma expansion in acute intracerebral hemorrhage. Eur Neurol 2013; 70(3–4):175–8.

37. Wong GK, Siu DY, Ahuja AT, et al. Comparisons of DSA and MR angiography with digital subtraction angiography in 151 patients with subacute spontaneous intracerebral hemorrhage. J Clin Neurosci 2010;17(5):601–5.

38. Takaoka H, Hashimoto A, Nogi S, et al. A case of granulomatosis with polyangiitis (Wegener's granulomatosis) manifested with asymptomatic intracerebral hemorrhage. Nihon Rinsho Meneki Gakkai Kaishi 2013;36(1):58–61.

39. Sumiya T. Hypertensive intracerebral hemorrhage due to autonomic dysreflexia in a young man with cervical cord injury. J UOEH 2013;35(2):159–64.

40. Teive HA, Ruschel E, Munhoz RP. Spontaneous intracerebral hemorrhage in Urbach-Wiethe disease. Neurology 2013;80(18):1720–1.

41. Kamel H, Navi BB, Hemphill JC 3rd. A rule to identify patients who require magnetic resonance imaging after intracerebral hemorrhage. Neurocrit Care 2013; 18(1):59–63.

42. Fuentes B, Martinez-Sanchez P, Raya PG, et al. Cerebral venous sinus thrombosis associated with cerebral hemorrhage: is anticoagulant treatment safe? Neurologist 2011;17(4):208–10.

43. Rodriguez-Luna D, Pineiro S, Rubiera M, et al. Impact of blood pressure changes and course on hematoma growth in acute intracerebral hemorrhage. Eur J Neurol 2013;20(9):1277–83.

44. Sakamoto Y, Koga M, Yamagami H, et al. Systolic blood pressure after intravenous antihypertensive treatment and clinical outcomes in hyperacute intracerebral hemorrhage: the stroke acute management with urgent risk-factor assessment and improvement-intracerebral hemorrhage study. Stroke 2013;44(7):1846–51.

45. Anderson CS, Heeley E, Huang Y, et al. Rapid blood-pressure lowering in patients with acute intracerebral hemorrhage. N Engl J Med 2013;368(25): 2355–65.

46. Butcher KS, Jeerakathil T, Hill M, et al. The intracerebral hemorrhage acutely decreasing arterial pressure trial. Stroke 2013;44(3):620–6.

47. Frontera JA. Blood pressure in intracerebral hemorrhage–how low should we go? N Engl J Med 2013;368(25):2426–7.

48. Honner SK, Singh A, Cheung PT, et al. Emergency department control of blood pressure in intracerebral hemorrhage. J Emerg Med 2011;41(4):355–61.

49. Sarode R, Matevosyan K, Bhagat R, et al. Rapid warfarin reversal: a 3-factor prothrombin complex concentrate and recombinant factor VIIa cocktail for intracerebral hemorrhage. J Neurosurg 2012;116(3):491–7.

50. Mayer SA, Brun NC, Begtrup K, et al. Efficacy and safety of recombinant activated factor VII for acute intracerebral hemorrhage. N Engl J Med 2008; 358(20):2127–37.

51. James RF, Palys V, Lomboy JR, et al. The role of anticoagulants, antiplatelet agents, and their reversal strategies in the management of intracerebral hemorrhage. Neurosurg Focus 2013;34(5):E6.

52. Campbell PG, Yadla S, Sen AN, et al. Emergency reversal of clopidogrel in the setting of spontaneous intracerebral hemorrhage. World Neurosurg 2011; 76(1–2):100–4 [discussion: 59–60].

53. Broderick JP. Evidence against rapid reversal of antiplatelet medications in acute intracerebral hemorrhage. Neurology 2009;72(16):1376–7.

54. Fan JS, Huang HH, Chen YC, et al. Emergency department neurologic deterioration in patients with spontaneous intracerebral hemorrhage: incidence, predictors, and prognostic significance. Acad Emerg Med 2012;19(2):133–8.

55. Sun W, Pan W, Kranz PG, et al. Predictors of late neurological deterioration after spontaneous intracerebral hemorrhage. Neurocrit Care 2013;19(3):299–305.

56. Maas MB, Rosenberg NF, Kosteva AR, et al. Surveillance neuroimaging and neurologic examinations affect care for intracerebral hemorrhage. Neurology 2013;81(2):107–12.

57. Kirkman MA, Smith M. Supratentorial intracerebral hemorrhage: a review of the underlying pathophysiology and its relevance for multimodality neuromonitoring in neurointensive care. J Neurosurg Anesthesiol 2013;25(3):228–39.

58. Diringer MN, Edwards DF. Admission to a neurologic/neurosurgical intensive care unit is associated with reduced mortality rate after intracerebral hemorrhage. Crit Care Med 2001;29(3):635–40.

59. Burns JD, Green DM, Lau H, et al. The effect of a neurocritical care service without a dedicated neuro-ICU on quality of care in intracerebral hemorrhage. Neurocrit Care 2013;18(3):305–12.

60. Maas MB, Nemeth AJ, Rosenberg NF, et al. Delayed intraventricular hemorrhage is common and worsens outcomes in intracerebral hemorrhage. Neurology 2013;80(14):1295–9.

61. Diringer MN, Edwards DF, Zazulia AR. Hydrocephalus: a previously unrecognized predictor of poor outcome from supratentorial intracerebral hemorrhage. Stroke 1998;29(7):1352–7.

62. Kamel H, Hemphill JC 3rd. Characteristics and sequelae of intracranial hypertension after intracerebral hemorrhage. Neurocrit Care 2012;17(2):172–6.

63. Tian Y, Wang Z, Jia Y, et al. Intracranial pressure variability predicts short-term outcome after intracerebral hemorrhage: a retrospective study. J Neurol Sci 2013;330(1–2):38–44.

64. Ye H, Su Y. Hemodynamic effects of mannitol infusion in patients with acute intracerebral hemorrhage. Acta Cir Bras 2013;28(2):106–11.

65. Christensen MC, Broderick J, Vincent C, et al. Global differences in patient characteristics, case management and outcomes in intracerebral hemorrhage: the Factor Seven for Acute Hemorrhagic Stroke (FAST) trial. Cerebrovasc Dis 2009;28(1):55–64.

66. Volbers B, Wagner I, Willfarth W, et al. Intraventricular fibrinolysis does not increase perihemorrhagic edema after intracerebral hemorrhage. Stroke 2013; 44(2):362–6.

67. Yeatts SD, Palesch YY, Moy CS, et al. High dose deferoxamine in intracerebral hemorrhage (HI-DEF) trial: rationale, design, and methods. Neurocrit Care 2013; 19(2):257–66.
68. Mendelow AD, Gregson BA, Fernandes HM, et al. Early surgery versus initial conservative treatment in patients with spontaneous supratentorial intracerebral haematomas in the International Surgical Trial in Intracerebral Haemorrhage (STICH): a randomised trial. Lancet 2005;365(9457):387–97.
69. Mendelow AD, Gregson BA, Rowan EN, et al. Early surgery versus initial conservative treatment in patients with spontaneous supratentorial lobar intracerebral haematomas (STICH II): a randomised trial. Lancet 2013;382(9890):397–408.
70. Rashid HU, Amin R, Rahman A, et al. Correlation between intracerebral hemorrhage score and surgical outcome of spontaneous intracerebral hemorrhage. Bangladesh Med Res Counc Bull 2013;39(1):1–5.
71. Degos V, Westbroek EM, Lawton MT, et al. Perioperative management of coagulation in nontraumatic intracerebral hemorrhage. Anesthesiology 2013;119(1): 218–27.
72. Hayes SB, Benveniste RJ, Morcos JJ, et al. Retrospective comparison of craniotomy and decompressive craniectomy for surgical evacuation of nontraumatic, supratentorial intracerebral hemorrhage. Neurosurg Focus 2013;34(5):E3.
73. Heuts SG, Bruce SS, Zacharia BE, et al. Decompressive hemicraniectomy without clot evacuation in dominant-sided intracerebral hemorrhage with ICP crisis. Neurosurg Focus 2013;34(5):E4.
74. Takeuchi S, Takasato Y, Masaoka H, et al. Decompressive craniectomy with hematoma evacuation for large hemispheric hypertensive intracerebral hemorrhage. Acta Neurochir Suppl 2013;118:277–9.
75. Chen CH, Lee HC, Chuang HC, et al. Transsylvian-transinsular approach for the removal of basal ganglia hemorrhage under a modified intracerebral hemorrhage score. J Craniofac Surg 2013;24(4):1388–92.
76. Burgner J, Swaney PJ, Lathrop RA, et al. Debulking from within: a robotic steerable cannula for intracerebral hemorrhage evacuation. IEEE Trans Biomed Eng 2013;60(9):2567–75.
77. Morgan T, Zuccarello M, Narayan R, et al. Preliminary findings of the minimally-invasive surgery plus rtPA for intracerebral hemorrhage evacuation (MISTIE) clinical trial. Acta Neurochir Suppl 2008;105:147–51.
78. Mullen MT, Kasner SE, Messe SR. Seizures do not increase in-hospital mortality after intracerebral hemorrhage in the nationwide inpatient sample. Neurocrit Care 2013;19(1):19–24.
79. Claassen J, Jette N, Chum F, et al. Electrographic seizures and periodic discharges after intracerebral hemorrhage. Neurology 2007;69(13):1356–65.
80. Naidech AM, Maas MB, Liotta EM, et al. Re: Confounding by indication in retrospective studies of intracerebral hemorrhage: antiepileptic treatment and mortality. Neurocrit Care 2013;18(2):285–6.
81. Naidech AM, Garg RK, Liebling S, et al. Anticonvulsant use and outcomes after intracerebral hemorrhage. Stroke 2009;40(12):3810–5.
82. Popescu D, Laza C, Mergeani A, et al. Lead electrocardiogram changes after supratentorial intracerebral hemorrhage. Maedica (Buchar) 2012;7(4):290–4.
83. Inamasu J, Ito K, Sugimoto K, et al. Cardiac wall motion abnormality associated with spontaneous intracerebral hemorrhage. Int J Cardiol 2013;168(2):1667–9.
84. Yaghi S, Moore P, Ray B, et al. Predictors of tracheostomy in patients with spontaneous intracerebral hemorrhage. Clin Neurol Neurosurg 2013;115(6): 695–8.

85. Roch A, Michelet P, Jullien AC, et al. Long-term outcome in intensive care unit survivors after mechanical ventilation for intracerebral hemorrhage. Crit Care Med 2003;31(11):2651–6.

86. Elmer J, Hou P, Wilcox SR, et al. Acute respiratory distress syndrome after spontaneous intracerebral hemorrhage*. Crit Care Med 2013;41(8):1992–2001.

87. Junttila E, Ala-Kokko T, Ohtonen P, et al. Neurogenic pulmonary edema in patients with nontraumatic intracerebral hemorrhage: predictors and association with outcome. Anesth Analg 2013;116(4):855–61.

88. Alsumrain M, Melillo N, Debari VA, et al. Predictors and outcomes of pneumonia in patients with spontaneous intracerebral hemorrhage. J Intensive Care Med 2013;28(2):118–23.

89. Lee JS, Jwa CS, Yi HJ, et al. Impact of early enteral nutrition on in-hospital mortality in patients with hypertensive intracerebral hemorrhage. J Korean Neurosurg Soc 2010;48(2):99–104.

90. Sykora M, Diedler J, Poli S, et al. Autonomic shift and increased susceptibility to infections after acute intracerebral hemorrhage. Stroke 2011;42(5):1218–23.

91. Kiphuth IC, Staykov D, Kohrmann M, et al. Early administration of low molecular weight heparin after spontaneous intracerebral hemorrhage. A safety analysis. Cerebrovasc Dis 2009;27(2):146–50.

92. Kuramatsu JB, Gerner S, Lucking H, et al. Anemia is an independent prognostic factor in intracerebral hemorrhage: an observational cohort study. Crit Care 2013;17(4):R148.

93. Sheth KN, Gilson AJ, Chang Y, et al. Packed red blood cell transfusion and decreased mortality in intracerebral hemorrhage. Neurosurgery 2011;68(5):1286–92.

94. Cho DY, Chen CC, Lee WY, et al. A new modified intracerebral hemorrhage score for treatment decisions in basal ganglia hemorrhage–a randomized trial. Crit Care Med 2008;36(7):2151–6.

95. Hemphill JC 3rd, Bonovich DC, Besmertis L, et al. The ICH score: a simple, reliable grading scale for intracerebral hemorrhage. Stroke 2001;32(4):891–7.

96. Ruiz-Sandoval JL, Chiquete E, Romero-Vargas S, et al. Grading scale for prediction of outcome in primary intracerebral hemorrhages. Stroke 2007;38(5):1641–4.

97. Parry-Jones AR, Abid KA, Di Napoli M, et al. Accuracy and clinical usefulness of intracerebral hemorrhage grading scores: a direct comparison in a UK population. Stroke 2013;44(7):1840–5.

98. Zahuranec DB, Morgenstern LB, Sanchez BN, et al. Do-not-resuscitate orders and predictive models after intracerebral hemorrhage. Neurology 2010;75(7):626–33.

99. Rost NS, Smith EE, Chang Y, et al. Prediction of functional outcome in patients with primary intracerebral hemorrhage: the FUNC score. Stroke 2008;39(8):2304–9.

100. Galbois A, Boelle PY, Hainque E, et al. Prediction of evolution toward brain death upon admission to ICU in comatose patients with spontaneous intracerebral hemorrhage using simple signs. Transpl Int 2013;26(5):517–26.

101. Herweh C, Prager E, Sykora M, et al. Cerebral atrophy is an independent risk factor for unfavorable outcome after spontaneous supratentorial intracerebral hemorrhage. Stroke 2013;44(4):968–71.

102. Kiphuth IC, Huttner HB, Dorfler A, et al. Doppler pulsatility index in spontaneous intracerebral hemorrhage. Eur Neurol 2013;70(3–4):133–8.

103. Lee JY, King C, Stradling D, et al. Influence of hematoma location on acute mortality after intracerebral hemorrhage. J Neuroimaging 2014;24(2):131–6.

104. Skolarus LE, Morgenstern LB, Zahuranec DB, et al. Acute care and long-term mortality among elderly patients with intracerebral hemorrhage who undergo chronic life-sustaining procedures. J Stroke Cerebrovasc Dis 2013;22(1):15–21.

105. Jain A, Jain M, Bellolio MF, et al. Is early DNR a self-fulfilling prophecy for patients with spontaneous intracerebral hemorrhage? Neurocrit Care 2013;19(3): 342–6.

106. Gathier CS, Algra A, Rinkel GJ, et al. Long-term outcome after anticoagulation-associated intracerebral haemorrhage with or without restarting antithrombotic therapy. Cerebrovasc Dis 2013;36(1):33–7.

107. Kim-Tenser M, Mack WJ. Anticoagulation in the setting of intracerebral hemorrhage: controversies in resuming therapy. World Neurosurg 2014;81(5–6): 669–70.

108. Amarenco P, Bogousslavsky J, Callahan A 3rd, et al. High-dose atorvastatin after stroke or transient ischemic attack. N Engl J Med 2006;355(6):549–59.

109. Hackam DG, Woodward M, Newby LK, et al. Statins and intracerebral hemorrhage: collaborative systematic review and meta-analysis. Circulation 2011; 124(20):2233–42.

110. Winkler J, Shoup JP, Czap A, et al. Long-term improvement in outcome after intracerebral hemorrhage in patients treated with statins. J Stroke Cerebrovasc Dis 2013;22(8):e541–5.

111. Jia W, Zhou L. Effect of 20 mg/day atorvastatin: recurrent stroke survey in Chinese ischemic stroke patients with prior intracranial hemorrhage. J Clin Neurol 2013;9(3):139–43.

Treatment of Subarachnoid Hemorrhage

Amanda K. Raya, MD, Michael N. Diringer, MD*

KEYWORDS

- Subarachnoid hemorrhage • Vasospasm • Delayed cerebral ischemia • Aneurysm
- Transcranial Doppler ultrasonography

KEY POINTS

- Subarachnoid hemorrhage is typically caused by a ruptured intracranial aneurysm and presents with a sudden severe, headache often accompanied by syncope, nausea, and vomiting.
- Initial management includes airway assessment, blood pressure control, treatment of pain, and noncontrast computed tomography (CT), followed by urgent catheter or CT angiography.
- To reduce the risk of delayed cerebral ischemia (DCI), all patients should be treated with nimodipine and be maintained in a euvolemic state in the days after hemorrhage.
- The development of narrowing of large cerebral vessels (vasospasm) can be detected with transcranial Doppler ultrasonography, CT, or conventional angiography. Vasospasm is closely correlated with DCI, but each can occur independently.
- DCI can be treated with combinations of blood pressure or cardiac output augmentation, angioplasty of proximal vasospastic vessels, and selective intra-arterial infusions of vasodilators.

INTRODUCTION

Nontraumatic subarachnoid hemorrhage (SAH) typically presents as a sudden severe headache, often described as "the worst headache of my life." Consciousness may be impaired, but focal neurologic deficits are uncommon. The incidence of SAH ranges from 10 to 18 per 100,000 people.[1] It often occurs in middle-aged patients and has a female predominance.[2] Of all spontaneous SAHs, 80% are the result of the rupture of an intracranial aneurysm, 15% do not have a bleeding source identified, and the remainder are owing to a myriad of other causes, mostly vascular malformations, but also vasculitis or posterior reversible vasoconstriction syndrome. Genetic factors seem to play a role in some families.

Disclosures: None.

Neurocritical Care Section, Department of Neurology, Washington University School of Medicine, 660 South Euclid Avenue, Campus Box 8111, St Louis, MO 63110, USA

* Corresponding author.

E-mail address: diringerm@wustl.edu

Crit Care Clin 30 (2014) 719–733

http://dx.doi.org/10.1016/j.ccc.2014.06.004

0749-0704/14/$ – see front matter © 2014 Elsevier Inc. All rights reserved.

criticalcare.theclinics.com

Intracranial berry (ie, saccular) aneurysms are typically found near the circle of Willis at the branching points of large cerebral arteries. Hemodynamic stress at arterial branching sites and inflammation seem to contribute to aneurysm formation. About 2% to 5% of the population harbor intracranial aneurysms.[3] Although aneurysms are thought to develop over many years, cases of rapid growth in size do occur. They frequently arise off the internal carotid artery at the take-off of the anterior and posterior communicating arteries and middle cerebral artery. Relatively few occur in the posterior circulation. Risk factors for aneurysmal rupture include smoking, hypertension, alcohol use, and having first-degree relatives with SAH.[4,5] Autosomal-dominant polycystic kidney disease is the most common heritable disorder to increase the risk for SAH; others include connective tissue disorders.

PATIENT EVALUATION

The classical clinical triad for presentation of SAH includes sudden severe headache, syncope, and vomiting. Other common symptoms include nausea, photophobia, and altered consciousness. Focal neurologic deficits occur in about 10% of patients. They can be owing to aneurysmal compression of a cranial nerve (typically a posterior communicating artery aneurysm compressing the third nerve producing ptosis, a dilated pupil, and limited medial and vertical gaze). More ominous are focal deficits owing to thick subarachnoid clots or parenchymal hematoma. Blood released under high pressure may directly cause damage to local tissues. Additionally, the vessel rupture produces an increase in intracranial pressure (ICP) that approaches arterial pressure and cerebral perfusion falls to nil. If hemorrhage stops and the acute rise in ICP is transient, it can result in nausea, vomiting, and syncope; if the high pressure is sustained, it is uniformly fatal. Exposure of the meninges to blood causes irritation resulting in photophobia, neck stiffness, and eventually back pain. Blood pressure is frequently elevated, which may increase the risk of re-rupture.

Initial Stabilization

Initial management should focus on airway management in comatose patients and blood pressure control to stabilize the patient, with the goal of obtaining a computed tomography (CT) scan as soon as possible (**Box 1**).

Patients may be unable to protect their airway and require intubation for multiple reasons, including hydrocephalus, seizure, or sedation. In addition, elective intubation may be necessary in agitated patients to safely and expeditiously perform cerebral angiography.

To reduce the risk of rebleeding before the aneurysm is secured, blood pressure should be maintained at the patients baseline levels or, if unknown, a mean arterial blood pressure of less than about 110 mm Hg. Effective pain control may be sufficient to manage blood pressure; otherwise short-acting intravenous medications (eg,

---

Box 1
Initial stabilization and evaluation

Airway assessment in comatose patients

Control hypertension

Treat headache

Noncontrast CT scan as soon as possible

Lumbar puncture if CT negative and suspicion high

labetalol and hydralazine) are preferred (**Table 1**). Alternatively, continuous infusions of calcium channel blockers (eg, nicardipine) can be effective, especially in patients with refractory hypertension. Cerebral vasodilators such as nitrates should be avoided because they can raise the ICP. If acute hydrocephalus is present, then management of blood pressure should be mitigated until a ventricular drain has been placed. After the aneurysm is secured, the blood pressure goals should be liberalized. This permissive hypertension may help to augment cerebral perfusion should delayed cerebral ischemia (DCI) develop.

Pain control is best achieved with judicious use of short-acting intravenous medications to avoid oversedation. Often, opiates are needed to be effective. Long-acting agents should be used with caution because their sedatives effects are difficult to distinguish from the development of hydrocephalus.

DIAGNOSIS
SAH

The preferred diagnostic procedure to identify the presence of SAH is noncontrast CT. In the first 12 hours, blood will be apparent on CT scan in nearly 100% of cases; over the first 24 hours, this value drops to 95% to 99%.[6,7] Although magnetic resonance imaging (MRI) may be as sensitive as CT within the first 1 or 2 days, it is usually logistically much more difficult to obtain. Two or more days after the ictus, MRI with fluid-attenuated inversion recovery or susceptibility weighted imaging sequences may be more sensitive.[8,9] If a diagnostic CT and/or MRI are negative and clinical suspicion is high, a lumbar puncture should be performed. Although the presence of a large number of red blood cells in the fluid is suggestive of SAH, it is frequently owing to a traumatic tap. A more definitive test is to evaluate the fluid for xanthochromia using spectrophotometric analysis. If the results are equivocal, then vascular imaging to look for an aneurysm may be considered.

Identification of Bleeding Source

Until recently, conventional digital subtraction angiography was considered the best test to elucidate an aneurysmal source of hemorrhage. More recently, CT angiography (CTA) has come into regular use but may miss small aneurysms. The sensitivity and specificity for CTA depends on the modality and experience of the reader and compared with conventional angiography is respectively, 90% to 97% and 93% to 100%. Most of the aneurysms missed are less than 4 mm.[10,11] MRI, magnetic resonance angiography, or CTA may also help with operative planning. If cerebral angiography fails to find an aneurysm, it should be repeated in a few days, because an aneurysm missed on the initial angiogram may be identified.

In 10% to 15% of SAH cases, an aneurysm or other cause of hemorrhage is not identified. The majority of these patients fit into the syndrome of perimesencepahlic nonaneurysmal SAH. In this case, the blood is only present in the basal cisterns and is thought to arise from venous rather than arterial bleeding. Their course is usually

Table 1			
Medications for blood pressure control on presentation			
	Dose	Mechanism of Action	Side Effects
Labetalol	5–20 mg	Alpha 1 and beta blocker	Bradycardia
Hydralazine	5–20 mg	Vasodilator	Tachycardia, headache, and flushing
Nicardipine	2–20 mg/h	Dihydropyridine calcium channel blocker	Headache, flushing, and peripheral edema

benign, without risk of rebleeding. DCI, vasospasm, and hydrocephalus can occur in these patients, although it is rare.

Clinical Grading Scales

There are 3 SAH grading scales that are well known and typically assigned at presentation. Each of the 3 scales was created for a different reason and none are strongly correlated with outcome. The Hunt and Hess scale was created in 1986 to help stratify patients based on surgical risk. It is easy to administer, well known, and has some predictive value for outcome. However, the categories may overlap and patients with poor grades can still have good outcomes.[12] The World Federation of Neurosurgeons scale was created in 1988 based on the Glasgow Coma Scale to help standardize assessment. It is easy to administer but reviews are mixed on how well each stage correlates with outcome.[13] The modified Fisher scale was created from the Fisher scale to better predict cerebral vasospasm based on CT characteristics in 2006. It does show an increase in vasospasm risk in the worst grade[14] and therefore is the most used for predicting DCI.

TREATMENT OF THE ANEURYSM

Aneurysms can be treated with surgical clipping or endovascular coiling. The choice of which treatment to perform is based on the location and shape of the aneurysm (neck to dome ratio), as well as the type of patient. Aneurysms in the middle cerebral artery region or in tortuous vessels are typically surgically clipped because of the difficulty in reaching the aneurysm through endovascular methods. Aneurysms that are deep in the brain or in the posterior circulation are better suited for endovascular coiling. Aneurysms in patients with multiple comorbidities are often treated with endovascular coiling. The International Subarachnoid Trial was a landmark study that randomly assigned aneurysms with clinical equipoise to clipping or coiling. Patients who had their aneurysms coiled had lower mortality and disability (7% absolute risk reduction of poor outcome) but a greater risk of rebleeding.[11,15] Typically, patients who have their aneurysm coiled require follow-up vascular imaging after 6 to 12 months to identify any inadequate occlusion and provide retreatment if coil compaction and recannulation of the aneurysm occurred.[16]

COMPLICATIONS
Seizures

It is not uncommon for seizurelike activity to occur at the time of hemorrhage. Whether these represent true seizures or motor posturing owing to elevated ICP is uncertain. Several studies have shown that there is no correlation between seizure activity at the time of aneurysm rupture and long-term epilepsy.

The risk of clinical seizures during hospitalization is low, at about 2%. However, in the minority of patients who have impaired consciousness, nonconvulsive status epilepticus is increasingly being found.[17] This has led to frequent use of continuous electroencephalographic monitoring in comatose patients. Based on data from the International Subarachnoid Trial, the risk of seizures after discharge is greater among patients who had their aneurysm treated surgically and can occur in up to 10% of patients.[18]

In patients who will have their aneurysms surgically repaired and have not had a seizure, most practitioners administer a short (3- to 7-day) course of prophylactic anticonvulsants. Patients who undergo coiling are not given prophylactic anticonvulsants in many centers. After a retrospective review that found that use of phenytoin after SAH was associated with worse long-term outcomes, leviratacetem has become the preferred agent for prophylaxis.[19] Patients who have had a seizure tend to be kept on anticonvulsants for one to several months.

Rebleeding

Rebleeding can be a devastating complication of SAH. In the first 24 hours, 4% to 15% of patients will rebleed; the risk of rebleeding decreases over the next 2 weeks. Administration of antifibrinolytics, early aneurysm repair, and blood pressure control are employed to reduce the chances of rebleeding.

Prolonged use of antifibrinolytics reduces the risk of rebleeding, but is also associated with increased ischemic events, negating any beneficial effects.[20] More recent studies of short-term use of antifibrinolytics ($\leq$3 days) suggest that rebleeding can be reduced without more risk of ischemia; thus they may be administered if aneurysm repair will be delayed. An ongoing multicenter, prospective, randomized, open-label trial is underway to determine whether a short-term antifibrinolytic leads to better functional outcome.[21]

Diagnostic CTA or catheter angiography should be performed as soon as possible, so that surgery or coiling can be undertaken and the aneurysm secured. The goal is to have the aneurysm repaired in less than 24 hours from presentation. Again, patients with unsecured aneurysms should have their blood pressure maintained in their normal range, or, if unknown, below a mean blood pressure of about 110 mm Hg.

Hydrocephalus

Hydrocephalus can complicate the SAH shortly after hemorrhage or it can develop in a delayed fashion. Acute hydrocephalus is evident on presentation or manifested by a progressive worsening of mental status within the first 1 to 3 days. On the initial CT scan, many patients exhibit radiographic hydrocephalus (which is based on the bicaudate index), but may be asymptomatic. About 20% develop symptomatic hydrocephalus and require placement of an external ventricular drain through a burr hole in the skull.[22] This fluid is allowed to drain until the patient's aneurysm is secured and patient is more stable. In about 40%, of cases hydrocephalus resolves and placement of a permanent shunt is not required. About 14% to 23% of all SAH patients, or 60% of those patients with an external ventricular drain, develop chronic hydrocephalus and require permanent cerebrospinal fluid (CSF) diversion.[23–27] Patients without acute hydrocephalus can develop delayed hydrocephalus weeks after hemorrhage, but this is rare. Older age, thicker blood clot in the subarachnoid space, increased ventricular size, and worse clinical grade are predictive of the need for placement of a permanent shunt.[24,28]

Cardiac

Cardiovascular disturbances after SAH range from minor disturbances in cardiac rate and rhythm to congestive heart failure and cardiogenic shock. Sinus arrhythmia, peaked T waves, T wave inversions, ST segment depressions or elevations, and prolongation of the QT interval are commonly seen on an electrocardiogram.[29] More significant rhythm disturbances are infrequent. Cardiac enzymes are elevated in 20% to 30% of patients, reflecting a catecholamine-related myocardial injury and a hypercontractile state rather than a lack of coronary blood flow.[30,31] Still, in patients with coronary artery disease, cardiac ischemia must be considered. Although the mean troponin value is typically low, some patients can have elevations of greater than 10.[32] In general, beta-blocking agents are administered to patients with elevated cardiac enzymes.

Echocardiography may be useful to help distinguish cardiac ischemia from catecholamine-induced cardiac injury and helps to assess cardiac function. Patients with changes on an electrocardiogram or elevated enzymes are more likely to have echocardiographic changes. Left ventricular dysfunction with wall motion abnormalities or a classic Takotsubo cardiomyopathy with apical ballooning are common echocardiographic findings. Takotsubo cardiomyopathy, so called owing to its similar shape on an echocardiogram to a Japanese "octopus pot," is more commonly found in those with a poor grade of SAH and elevated cardiac enzymes and is associated with an increased risk of cerebral vasospasm.[33,34] Acute cardiomyopathies may require aggressive management using standard approaches to management of congestive heart failure, including judicious diuresis, inotropic agents, and, in extreme cases, intra-aortic balloon pumps. Cardiac dysfunction, even if severe, typically begins to resolve within several days.

Cardiac dysfunction is frequently complicated by pulmonary edema attributed to both cardiac and neurogenic causes. Pulmonary edema owing to a neurologic injury is typically managed the same way as other causes of pulmonary edema. When mechanical ventilation is needed, hypercarbia should be avoided owing to its detrimental effect on ICP. Similarly, nitroglycerin and nitroprusside should be avoided because their venovasodilatory effects can markedly elevate ICP. Because cardiomyopathy occurs early after hemorrhage before the period of vasospasm, lower blood pressures may be tolerated.

Fever

Fever is associated with worse outcomes, including increased disability and cognitive impairment outcomes from SAH.[35] It is likely a component of the systemic inflammatory response caused by SAH. Initially, all fevers should be investigated as a possible infection. Antipyretics (typically acetaminophen and ibuprofen) may be effective, but in some cases additional measures are needed including ice packs, cooling blankets, and other surface or intravascular cooling devices.[36,37] As fever is treated, shivering can occur, increasing metabolic demand and heat production. Shivering should be treated; options include surface counterwarming, meperidine, buspirone, dexmedetomidine, and potentially intravenous magnesium infusion.

Hyponatremia

Hyponatremia complicates the course of about one third of SAH patients and has been associated in past and contemporary studies with poorer outcomes. A number of studies indicate that it is likely owing to a combination of cerebral salt wasting (excessive renal sodium and water excretion) and syndrome of inappropriate antidiuretic hormone (inappropriate renal water retention). In an attempt to avoid hyponatremia, SAH patients are administered isotonic fluids. Because of its potential for exacerbating cerebral edema, hyponatremia is usually treated at very mild levels. Because hypovolemia associated with fluid restriction may increase the risk for DCI, hyponatremia after SAH is not treated with fluid restriction, but with oral free water restriction and administration of mildly hypertonic fluids such as 1.5% or 2% sodium chloride.[38] Use of fludrocortisone or hydrocortisone may help with diuresis and help to reduce hyponatremia.[39,40] Vasopressin receptor agonists are effective in correcting hyponatremia, but they must be used with caution because they can cause a brisk diuresis and hypovolemia.

Vasospasm and DCI

It has long been recognized that some SAH patients deteriorate neurologically several days after hemorrhage. More than 5 years ago, these deteriorations were linked with arterial narrowing and later with reduced cerebral blood flow (CBF). Although arterial narrowing is currently referred to as "vasospasm," the clinical syndrome is now referred to as "delayed cerebral ischemia" (DCI). DCI is defined as the occurrence of neurologic deterioration that is not owing to other causes, or the evidence of a new infarct on CT imaging performed more than 72 hours after aneurysm rupture (**Box 2, Tables 2** and **3**).[41] Infarction is a major complication of SAH because it has such a great impact on functional outcome. DCI peaks between days 3 and 14 and affects about 30% of patients. The risk of DCI is increased with a greater volume of SAH, intraventricular hemorrhage, poor clinical condition on admission, and a history of smoking.[42]

DCI may be caused by many factors, including arterial vasospasm, cortical spreading depression, inflammation, and intravascular microthrombosis. Vasospasm of large cerebral conducting vessels can be easily identified with angiography or transcranial Doppler ultrasonography (TCD) and is common in patients who develop DCI. Approximately 70% of patients develop evidence of vasospasm after SAH and somewhat fewer than half develop DCI. The release of oxygenated hemoglobin into the CSF initiates an inflammatory cascade that results initially in smooth muscle contraction and eventually in hypertrophy and fibrosis of the vessel walls. Arterial vasospasm may start appearing 3 days after rupture and reaches a peak in incidence and severity at 7 to 10 days.

DCI prophylaxis: euvolemia

Up to half of SAH patients treated with standard maintenance volume of fluids develop intravascular volume contraction. In older studies, fluid restriction to treat hyponatremia was associated with infarction and worse outcomes. In randomized, controlled trials, prophylactic hypervolemia did not improve CBF or clinical outcomes and was associated with an higher risk of cardiopulmonary complications.[43,44] Typically euvolemia is ensured by strict monitoring of fluids and replacement of urine output starting approximately 3 days after the initial SAH. Fludrocortisone or hydrocortisone may be helpful in patients with significant diuresis.[45] The use of pulmonary artery catheters and central venous pressure monitoring to direct fluid management is not currently recommended owing to potential complications and a lack of data to support effectiveness.

Box 2
Management of delayed cerebral ischemia (DCI)

Prophylaxis

- Nimodipine
- Maintenance of euvolemia
- Lumbar drainage

Symptomatic DCI

- Medical
  - Induced hypertension
  - Cardiac output augmentation
  - Transfusion
- Endovascular
  - Angioplasty
  - Intra-arterial vasodilators

Table 2
Definitions

Term	Large Vessel Narrowing	Clinical Symptoms	Infarction
Vasospasm	Identified on TCD, angiogram or CTA	May or may not be present	May or may not be present
DCI	May or may not be present	Must be present	May or may not be present, if present sufficient for diagnosis

Abbreviations: CTA, computed tomography angiography; TCD, transcranial Doppler ultrasonography.

DCI prophylaxis: calcium channel blockers

Nimodipine has been standard of care for SAH for almost 3 decades. In a recent meta-analysis, nimodipine had a relative risk reduction of poor outcome of 0.67 with a recommended dose of 60 mg every 4 hours for 3 weeks.[46] Nimodipine seems to exert its effect owing to its action on neuronal calcium channels; it does not reduce the rate of vasospasm even though it improves outcomes.

DCI prophylaxis: lumbar drains

Lumbar drains may wash out the blood from the subarachnoid space and, consequently, inflammatory mediators that could cause cerebral vasospasm. Recent studies have suggested that lumbar CSF drainage can prevent DCI.[47,48] Although it does not change the need for permanent CSF diversion, and the results for long-term outcomes are not robust, it has consistently shown a decrease in DCI and further studies are ongoing.

Diagnosing Vasospasm and DCI

Diagnosis and monitoring for clinically relevant vasospasm and DCI can be done several ways. Neurologic examinations are done multiple times per day (usually every 2 hours) to monitor for clinical signs of DCI. If a clinical examination deteriorates (a decrease of 2 points on the Glasgow Coma Scale or a new focal deficit), an evaluation for other causes (fever, metabolic disturbance, cerebral edema, or hydrocephalus) is indicated. Additional testing to corroborate a diagnosis of DCI (see below) may be undertaken or therapy initiated.

TCD

Some centers perform daily TCD to measure CBF velocity. As vessels narrow from vasospasm, CBF velocities rise (assuming CBF is unchanged). The threshold for mild vasospasm is considered greater than 120 cm/sec in the middle cerebral artery

Table 3
Management of common complications

Complication	Management
Seizures	Prophylactic anti-epileptics for 3–7 d
Rebleeding	Blood pressure control, early aneurysm treatment
Hydrocephalus	Extraventricular drainage
Cardiac dysfunction	Echocardiogram, euvolemia
Fever	Antipyretics, surface cooling, intravascular cooling
Hyponatremia	Hypertonic fluids

and greater than 200 cm/sec for severe vasospasm. Additional indicators include change in serial measurements of more than 50 cm/sec, or a Lindegaard index (ratio of middle cerebral artery to internal carotid artery velocity) of greater than 6. This technique is limited by its ability to evaluate only large proximal arteries, limited utility in the posterior circulation, and poor specificity.[49] Operator error and difficult temporal bone windows can make it unreliable. In combination with clinical examination, the majority of centers use serial TCD to judge which patients need further imaging with CT angiogram or conventional angiography.

CTA, CT perfusion, and angiography

Routine angiography during the critical phase of highest risk for DCI is another option for screening for vasospasm. More recently, CTA and CT perfusion have emerged as possible modalities to screen for and diagnose DCI and vasospasm. The combination of CTA findings for arterial narrowing and CBF with elevated mean transit time are the most accurate. These techniques are still evolving but recent studies publish sensitivities of 74% to 84% and specificity of 79% to 93%.[50,51]

DCI Management: Hemodynamic Augmentation

Induced hypertension

Treating DCI by elevating blood pressure has now become standard treatment for symptomatic patients. Its use in asymptomatic patients with evidence of vasospasm is controversial and is not recommended. There are case reports and case series that have shown that induced hypertension improves CBF and leads to neurologic improvement.[52,53] Norepinephrine and phenylephrine are the most common agents used. Blood pressure targets can be based on a percent increase above baseline blood pressure (typically beginning with a 10%–15% rise) or a target can be arbitrarily chosen. If there is no clinical response, vasopressors should be increased further. Once the patient improves, or further increases in blood pressure are considered imprudent, the target pressure is maintained for 1 to 3 days. CTA or cerebral angiography may be repeated to assess whether the vasospasm has abated and a trial of weaning therapy may be initiated. The blood pressure target is gradually lowered while closely monitoring with clinical examinations. Any deterioration should lead to a prompt increase in pressure. After another day or two, weaning should again be attempted. The use of induced hypertension is currently being tested in a multicenter, single-blinded, randomized, controlled trial.[54]

Augmenting cardiac output

There have been isolated reports of the use of inotropic agents to treat DCI.[55,56] It is generally reserved for patients who fail to respond to induced hypertension or have poor cardiac function. Dobutamine and milrinone are the most common inotropic agents employed for this indication.

Hemoglobin

Hemodilution for patients with DCI has been abandoned with the appreciation that the fall in hematocrit and thus arterial oxygen content lowers cerebral oxygen delivery. Additionally, anemia has been identified as a risk factor for DCI and poor outcome after SAH. Although retrospective studies point to risk associated with transfusion, a prospective study found that transfusion in anemic SAH patients was associated with improved brain oxygen delivery.[57] The current guidelines recommend transfusions to maintain hemoglobin concentration of greater than 8 to 10 g/dL and suggest that higher hemoglobin concentrations may be appropriate for patients with DCI.

DCI Management: Intra-arterial Treatment

Interventional therapies for DCI include transluminal angioplasty and infusion of intra-arterial vasodilators. Although some patients respond well to hemodynamic interventions, others do not respond to medical measures or cannot tolerate them owing to comorbidities. How long to wait until declaring hemodynamic interventions a failure is a matter of much discussion and few data exist, with recommendations ranging from 2 to 12 hours. Intra-arterial nimodipine, verapamil, nicardipine, and milrinone have all been shown to dilate blood vessels and augment CBF.[56,58,59] The duration of this response, however, seems to be a few hours. The effects of balloon angioplasty, on the other hand, are sustained. The use of angioplasty has been limited by its inability to reach distal vessels and risk of rupture associated with early balloon designs.[60] A prospective, randomized trial of prophylactic angioplasty in high-risk patients found it reduced DCI, but this was offset by complications owing to vessel rupture. Still, with improved balloon design, angioplasty is now routinely used in symptomatic patients.

PROGNOSIS

The overall mortality from SAH is 30% to 40%; about one half of patients die before they reach the hospital. Of the remainder, 25% die in the first 2 weeks.[61,62] Of the survivors, one half have a good recovery, yet studies show that survivors with good outcome still typically experience cognitive deficits in memory, executive function, and attention that impact their day-to-day living.[63]

Among other factors, poor prognosis is associated with advancing age, worsening neurologic grade, ruptured posterior circulation aneurysm, greater aneurysm size, more SAH, and most recently the Apo lipoprotein E ε4 allele.[64,65] Prognostication may be aided by electroencephalographic, although no specific pattern has been validated.[66] Repeat CT or MRI can be helpful to identify silent infarctions.

SUMMARY

Because one half of patients with aneurysmal SAH survive to reach the hospital, practitioners of neurocritical care continue to search for modalities to prevent, detect, and ameliorate the secondary complications of vasospasm and DCI that worsens diffuse brain injury and cognitive deficits that impact the long-term functioning of these patients.

REFERENCES

1. Ingall T, Asplund K, Mahonen M, et al. A multinational comparison of subarachnoid hemorrhage epidemiology in the WHO MONICA stroke study. Stroke 2000; 31(5):1054–61. Available at: http://stroke.ahajournals.org/cgi/doi/10.1161/01. STR.31.5.1054. Accessed April 18, 2014.
2. De Rooij NK, Linn FH, van der Plas JA, et al. Incidence of subarachnoid haemorrhage: a systematic review with emphasis on region, age, gender and time trends. J Neurol Neurosurg Psychiatry 2007;78:1365–72. Available at: http://www.pubmedcentral.nih.gov/articlerender.fcgi?artid=2095631&tool=pmcentrez&rendertype=abstract. Accessed April 12, 2014.
3. Rinkel GJ, Djibuti M, Algra A, et al. Prevalence and risk of rupture of intracranial aneurysms: a systematic review. Stroke 1998;29(1):251–6. Available at: http://stroke.ahajournals.org/cgi/doi/10.1161/01.STR.29.1.251. Accessed April 7, 2014.

4. Teasdale GM, Wardlaw JM, White PM, et al. The familial risk of subarachnoid haemorrhage. Brain 2005;128(Pt 7):1677–85. Available at: http://www.ncbi. nlm.nih.gov/pubmed/15817512. Accessed April 18, 2014.

5. Yahia AM, Suarez JI, Guterman LR, et al. Risk factors for subarachnoid hemorrhage. Neurosurgery 2001;49(3):607–13.

6. Sames TA, Storrow AB, Finkelstein JA, et al. Sensitivity of new-generation computed tomography in subarachnoid hemorrhage. Acad Emerg Med 1996; 3(1):16–20. Available at: http://www.ncbi.nlm.nih.gov/pubmed/8749962.

7. Cortnum S, Sørensen P, Jørgensen J. Determining the sensitivity of computed tomography scanning in early detection of subarachnoid hemorrhage. Neurosurgery 2010;66(5):900–3. Available at: http://journals.lww.com/neurosurgery/ Abstract/2010/05000/Determining_the_Sensitivity_of_Computed_Tomography.7. aspx. Accessed April 23, 2014.

8. Fiebach JB, Schellinger PD, Geletneky K, et al. MRI in acute subarachnoid haemorrhage; findings with a standardised stroke protocol. Neuroradiology 2004; 46(1):44–8. Available at: http://www.ncbi.nlm.nih.gov/pubmed/14655034. Accessed April 10, 2014.

9. Mitchell P, Wilkinson ID, Hoggard N, et al. Detection of subarachnoid haemorrhage with magnetic resonance imaging. J Neurol Neurosurg Psychiatry 2001; 70(2):205–11. Available at: http://www.pubmedcentral.nih.gov/articlerender. fcgi?artid=1737199&tool=pmcentrez&rendertype=abstract.

10. Teksam M, McKinney A, Casey S, et al. Multi-section CT angiography for detection of cerebral aneurysms. AJNR Am J Neuroradiol 2004;25(9):1485–92. Available at: http://www.ncbi.nlm.nih.gov/pubmed/15502126.

11. Molyneux A, Kerr R, Stratton I, et al. International Subarachnoid Aneurysm Trial (ISAT) of neurosurgical clipping versus endovascular coiling in 2143 patients with ruptured intracranial aneurysms: a randomized trial. J Stroke Cerebrovasc Dis 2002;11(6):304–14. Available at: http://www.ncbi.nlm.nih.gov/pubmed/ 17903891. Accessed April 13, 2014.

12. Aulmann C. Validation of the prognostic accuracy of neurosurgical admission scales after rupture of cerebral aneurysms. Zentralbl Neurochir 1998;59(3): 171–80 [in German].

13. Rosen DS, Macdonald RL. Grading of subarachnoid hemorrhage: modification of the world federation of neurosurgical societies scale on the basis of data for a large series of patients. Neurosurgery 2004;54(3):566–76. Available at: http://content. wkhealth.com/linkback/openurl?sid=WKPTLP:landingpage&an=00006123-20040 3000-00017. Accessed April 18, 2014.

14. Frontera J, Claassen J. Prediction of symptomatic vasospasm after subarachnoid hemorrhage: the modified fisher scale. Neurosurgery 2006;58(7):21–7. Available at: http://journals.lww.com/neurosurgery/Abstract/2006/07000/ Prediction_of_Symptomatic_Vasospasmafter.3.aspx. Accessed April 23, 2014.

15. Molyneux AJ, Kerr RS, Yu LM, et al. International subarachnoid aneurysm trial (ISAT) of neurosurgical clipping versus endovascular coiling in 2143 patients with ruptured intracranial aneurysms: a randomised comparison of effects on survival, dependency, seizures, rebleeding, subgroups, and aneurysm occlusion. Lancet 2005;366(9488):809–17. Available at: http://www.ncbi.nlm.nih. gov/pubmed/16139655.

16. Johnston SC, Higashida RT, Barrow DL, et al. Recommendations for the endovascular treatment of intracranial aneurysms: a statement for healthcare professionals from the committee on cerebrovascular imaging of the American Heart Association Council on Cardiovascular Radiology. Stroke 2002;33(10):2536–44.

Available at: http://stroke.ahajournals.org/cgi/doi/10.1161/01.STR.0000034708.
66191.7D. Accessed March 22, 2014.

17. Dennis L, Claassen J, Hirsch L. Nonconvulsive status epilepticus after subarachnoid hemorrhage. Neurosurgery 2002;51(5):1136–44. Available at: http://journals.lww.com/neurosurgery/Abstract/2002/11000/Nonconvulsive_Status_Epilepticus_after.6.aspx. Accessed April 23, 2014.

18. Hart Y, Sneade M, Birks J, et al. Epilepsy after subarachnoid hemorrhage: the frequency of seizures after clip occlusion or coil embolization of a ruptured cerebral aneurysm: results from the International Subarachnoid Aneurysm Trial. J Neurosurg 2011;115(6):1159–68. Available at: http://www.ncbi.nlm.nih.gov/pubmed/21819189. Accessed April 18, 2014.

19. Naidech AM, Kreiter KT, Janjua N, et al. Phenytoin exposure is associated with functional and cognitive disability after subarachnoid hemorrhage. Stroke 2005; 36(3):583–7. Available at: http://www.ncbi.nlm.nih.gov/pubmed/15662039. Accessed March 23, 2014.

20. Roos Y, Rinkel G. Antifibrinolytic therapy for aneurysmal subarachnoid haemorrhage. Stroke 2003;34(2):2308–9. Available at: http://onlinelibrary.wiley.com/doi/10.1002/14651858.CD001245/pdf/standard. Accessed April 23, 2014.

21. Germans MR, Post R, Coert BA, et al. Ultra-early tranexamic acid after subarachnoid hemorrhage (ULTRA): study protocol for a randomized controlled trial. Trials 2013;14:143. Available at: http://www.pubmedcentral.nih.gov/articlerender.fcgi?artid=3658919&tool=pmcentrez&rendertype=abstract. Accessed April 18, 2014.

22. Suarez-Rivera M. Acute hydrocephalus after subarachnoid hemorrhage. Surg Neurol 1998;49:563–5. Available at: http://www.sciencedirect.com/science/article/pii/S009030199700342X. Accessed April 23, 2014.

23. Vale FL, Bradley EL, Fisher WS. The relationship of subarachnoid hemorrhage and the need for postoperative shunting. J Neurosurg 1997;86(3):462–6. Available at: http://www.ncbi.nlm.nih.gov/pubmed/9046303.

24. Dorai Z, Hynan LS, Kopitnik TA, et al. Factors related to hydrocephalus after aneurysmal subarachnoid hemorrhage. Neurosurgery 2003;52(4):763–71. Available at: http://content.wkhealth.com/linkback/openurl?sid=WKPTLP:landingpage&an=00006123-200304000-00007. Accessed April 18, 2014.

25. Wright J, Huang C, Strbian D, et al. Diagnosis and management of acute cerebellar infarction. Stroke 2014;10:1–3 Strbian D, Sundararajan S, section editors. Available at: http://www.ncbi.nlm.nih.gov/pubmed/24558094. Accessed March 24, 2014.

26. O'Kelly CJ, Kulkarni AV, Austin PC, et al. Shunt-dependent hydrocephalus after aneurysmal subarachnoid hemorrhage: incidence, predictors, and revision rates. Clinical article. J Neurosurg 2009;111(5):1029–35. Available at: http://www.ncbi.nlm.nih.gov/pubmed/19361256. Accessed April 18, 2014.

27. Woernle CM, Winkler KM, Burkhardt JK, et al. Hydrocephalus in 389 patients with aneurysm-associated subarachnoid hemorrhage. J Clin Neurosci 2013; 20(6):824–6. Available at: http://www.ncbi.nlm.nih.gov/pubmed/23562295. Accessed April 18, 2014.

28. Yoshioka H, Inagawa T, Tokuda Y, et al. Chronic hydrocephalus in elderly patients following subarachnoid hemorrhage. Surg Neurol 2000;53(2):119–24 [discussion: 124–5]. Available at: http://www.ncbi.nlm.nih.gov/pubmed/10713188.

29. Lanzino G. Electrocardiographic abnormalities after nontraumatic subarachnoid hemorrhage. J Neurosurg 1994;6:156–62. Available at: http://journals.lww.com/jnsa/Abstract/1994/07000/Electrocardiographic_Abnormalities_After.2.aspx. Accessed April 23, 2014.

30. Gupte M, John S, Prabhakaran S, et al. Troponin elevation in subarachnoid hemorrhage does not impact in-hospital mortality. Neurocrit Care 2013;18(3): 368–73. Available at: http://www.ncbi.nlm.nih.gov/pubmed/23283601. Accessed April 22, 2014.

31. Jeon IC, Chang CH, Choi BY, et al. Cardiac troponin I elevation in patients with aneurysmal subarachnoid hemorrhage. J Korean Neurosurg Soc 2009;46(2): 99–102. Available at: http://www.pubmedcentral.nih.gov/articlerender.fcgi? artid=2744033&tool=pmcentrez&rendertype=abstract.

32. Naidech AM, Kreiter KT, Janjua N, et al. Cardiac troponin elevation, cardiovascular morbidity, and outcome after subarachnoid hemorrhage. Circulation 2005; 112(18):2851–6. Available at: http://www.ncbi.nlm.nih.gov/pubmed/16267258. Accessed April 5, 2014.

33. Lee V, Oh J, Mulvagh S, et al. Mechanisms in neurogenic stress cardiomyopathy after aneurysmal subarachnoid hemorrhage. Neurocrit Care 2006;5(3):243–9. Available at: http://link.springer.com/article/10.1385/NCC:5:3:243. Accessed April 23, 2014.

34. Kawai S, Susuki H, Yamaguchi H, et al. Ampulla cardiomyopathy Takotsubo cardiomyopathy: reversible left ventricular dysfunction with ST elevation. Jpn Circ J 2000;64:156–9.

35. Fernandez A, Schmidt JM, Claassen J, et al. Fever after subarachnoid hemorrhage: risk factors and impact on outcome. Neurology 2007;68(13):1013–9. Available at: http://www.ncbi.nlm.nih.gov/pubmed/17314332. Accessed April 22, 2014.

36. Diringer MN. Treatment of fever in the neurologic intensive care unit with a catheter-based heat exchange system. Crit Care Med 2004;32(2):559–64. Available at: http://www.ncbi.nlm.nih.gov/pubmed/14758179. Accessed April 5, 2014.

37. Hoedemaekers CW, Ezzahti M, Gerritsen A, et al. Comparison of cooling methods to induce and maintain normo- and hypothermia in intensive care unit patients: a prospective intervention study. Crit Care 2007;11(4):R91. Available at: http://www. pubmedcentral.nih.gov/articlerender.fcgi?artid=2206487&tool=pmcentrez& rendertype=abstract. Accessed March 30, 2014.

38. Wijdicks EF, Vermeulen M, Hijdra A, et al. Hyponatremia and cerebral infarction in patients with ruptured intracranial aneurysms: is fluid restriction harmful? Ann Neurol 1985;17(2):137–40.

39. Katayama Y, Haraoka J, Hirabayashi H, et al. A randomized controlled trial of hydrocortisone against hyponatremia in patients with aneurysmal subarachnoid hemorrhage. Stroke 2007;38(8):2373–5. Available at: http://www.ncbi.nlm.nih. gov/pubmed/17585086. Accessed April 22, 2014.

40. Mori T, Katayama Y, Kawamata T, et al. Improved efficiency of hypervolemic therapy with inhibition of natriuresis by fludrocortisone in patients with aneurysmal subarachnoid hemorrhage. J Neurosurg 1999;91(6):947–52. Available at: http://www.ncbi.nlm.nih.gov/pubmed/10584839.

41. Vergouwen MD, Vermeulen M, van Gijn J, et al. Definition of delayed cerebral ischemia after aneurysmal subarachnoid hemorrhage as an outcome event in clinical trials and observational studies: proposal of a multidisciplinary research group. Stroke 2010;41(10):2391–5. Available at: http://www.ncbi.nlm.nih.gov/ pubmed/20798370. Accessed October 21, 2013.

42. De Rooij NK, Rinkel GJ, Dankbaar JW, et al. Delayed cerebral ischemia after subarachnoid hemorrhage: a systematic review of clinical, laboratory, and radiological predictors. Stroke 2013;44(1):43–54. Available at: http://www.ncbi. nlm.nih.gov/pubmed/23250997. Accessed October 17, 2013.

43. Lennihan L, Mayer SA, Fink ME, et al. Effect of hypervolemic therapy on cerebral blood flow after subarachnoid hemorrhage: a randomized controlled trial. Stroke 2000;31(2):383–91. Available at: http://stroke.ahajournals.org/cgi/doi/10.1161/01.STR.31.2.383. Accessed April 15, 2014.

44. Egge A, Waterloo K, Sjøholm H. Prophylactic hyperdynamic postoperative fluid therapy after aneurysmal subarachnoid hemorrhage: a clinical, prospective, randomized, controlled study. Neurosurgery 2001;49(3):593–605. Available at: http://journals.lww.com/neurosurgery/Abstract/2001/09000/Prophylactic_Hyperdynamic_Postoperative_Fluid.12.aspx. Accessed April 23, 2014.

45. Moro N, Katayama Y, Kojima J, et al. Prophylactic management of excessive natriuresis with hydrocortisone for efficient hypervolemic therapy after subarachnoid hemorrhage. Stroke 2003;34(12):2807–11. Available at: http://www.ncbi.nlm.nih.gov/pubmed/14657545. Accessed April 22, 2014.

46. Dorhout Mees S. Calcium antagonists for aneurysmal subarachnoid haemorrhage. Stroke 2008;39:514–5. Available at: http://onlinelibrary.wiley.com/doi/10.1002/14651858.CD000277.pub2/full. Accessed April 23, 2014.

47. Kwon OY, Kim YJ, Kim YJ, et al. The utility and benefits of external lumbar CSF drainage after endovascular coiling on aneurysmal subarachnoid hemorrhage. J Korean Neurosurg Soc 2008;43(6):281–7. Available at: http://www.pubmedcentral.nih.gov/articlerender.fcgi?artid=2588254&tool=pmcentrez&rendertype=abstract.

48. Klimo P, Kestle JR, MacDonald JD, et al. Marked reduction of cerebral vasospasm with lumbar drainage of cerebrospinal fluid after subarachnoid hemorrhage. J Neurosurg 2004;100(2):215–24. Available at: http://www.ncbi.nlm.nih.gov/pubmed/15086227.

49. Suarez JI, Qureshi AI, Yahia AB. Symptomatic vasospasm diagnosis after subarachnoid hemorrhage: evaluation of transcranial Doppler ultrasound and cerebral angiography as related to compromised vascular distribution. Crit Care Med 2002;30(6):1348–55.

50. Greenberg ED, Gold R, Reichman M, et al. Diagnostic accuracy of CT angiography and CT perfusion for cerebral vasospasm: a meta-analysis. AJNR Am J Neuroradiol 2010;31(10):1853–60. Available at: http://www.pubmedcentral.nih.gov/articlerender.fcgi?artid=3130003&tool=pmcentrez&rendertype=abstract. Accessed April 22, 2014.

51. Dankbaar JW, de Rooij NK, Velthuis BK, et al. Diagnosing delayed cerebral ischemia with different CT modalities in patients with subarachnoid hemorrhage with clinical deterioration. Stroke 2009;40(11):3493–8. Available at: http://www.ncbi.nlm.nih.gov/pubmed/19762703. Accessed April 13, 2014.

52. Muizelaar J, Becker D. Induced hypertension for the treatment of cerebral ischemia after subarachnoid hemorrhage. Direct effect on cerebral blood flow. Surg Neurol 1986;25:317–25. Available at: http://www.sciencedirect.com/science/article/pii/0090301986902053. Accessed April 23, 2014.

53. Otsubo H, Takemae T, Inoue T. Normovolaemic induced hypertension therapy for cerebral vasospasm after subarachnoid haemorrhage. Acta Neurochir (Wien) 1990;103:18–26. Available at: http://link.springer.com/article/10.1007/BF01420187. Accessed April 23, 2014.

54. Gathier CS, van den Bergh WM, Slooter AJ, et al. HIMALAIA (Hypertension induction in the management of aneurysmal subArachnoid haemorrhage with secondary IschaemiA): a randomized single-blind controlled trial of induced hypertension vs. no induced hypertension in the treatment of delayed cerebral ischemia after subarachnoid hemorrhage. Int J Stroke 2014;9:375–80. Available

at: http://onlinelibrary.wiley.com/doi/10.1111/ijs.12055/full. Accessed April 23, 2014.

55. Rondeau N, Cinotti R, Rozec B, et al. Dobutamine-induced high cardiac index did not prevent vasospasm in subarachnoid hemorrhage patients: a random-ized controlled pilot study. Neurocrit Care 2012;17(2):183–90. Available at: http://www.ncbi.nlm.nih.gov/pubmed/22826137. Accessed April 22, 2014.

56. Fraticelli AT, Cholley BP, Losser MR, et al. Milrinone for the treatment of cerebral vasospasm after aneurysmal subarachnoid hemorrhage. Stroke 2008;39(3): 893–8. Available at: http://www.ncbi.nlm.nih.gov/pubmed/18239182. Accessed March 23, 2014.

57. Dhar R, Scalfani MT, Zazulia AR, et al. Comparison of induced hypertension, fluid bolus, and blood transfusion to augment cerebral oxygen delivery after subarach-noid hemorrhage. J Neurosurg 2012;116(3):648–56. Available at: http://www.pubmedcentral.nih.gov/articlerender.fcgi?artid=3763719&tool=pmcentrez&rendertype=abstract. Accessed March 21, 2014.

58. Romero CM, Morales D, Reccius A, et al. Milrinone as a rescue therapy for symptomatic refractory cerebral vasospasm in aneurysmal subarachnoid hem-orrhage. Neurocrit Care 2009;11(2):165–71. Available at: http://www.ncbi.nlm.nih.gov/pubmed/18202923. Accessed April 6, 2014.

59. Sehy JV, Holloway WE, Lin SP, et al. Improvement in angiographic cerebral vasospasm after intra-arterial verapamil administration. AJNR Am J Neuroradiol 2010;31(10):1923–8. Available at: http://www.ncbi.nlm.nih.gov/pubmed/20705701. Accessed April 22, 2014.

60. Polin RS, Coenen VA, Hansen CA, et al. Efficacy of transluminal angioplasty for the management of symptomatic cerebral vasospasm following aneurysmal subarachnoid hemorrhage. J Neurosurg 2000;92(2):284–90. Available at: http://www.ncbi.nlm.nih.gov/pubmed/10659016.

61. Nieuwkamp DJ, Setz LE, Algra A, et al. Changes in case fatality of aneurysmal subarachnoid haemorrhage over time, according to age, sex, and region: a meta-analysis. Lancet Neurol 2009;8(7):635–42. Available at: http://www.ncbi.nlm.nih.gov/pubmed/19501022. Accessed April 22, 2014.

62. Stegmayr B, Eriksson M, Asplund K. Declining mortality from subarachnoid hemorrhage: changes in incidence and case fatality from 1985 through 2000. Stroke 2004;35(9):2059–63. Available at: http://www.ncbi.nlm.nih.gov/pubmed/15272133. Accessed April 22, 2014.

63. Al-Khindi T, Macdonald RL, Schwizer TA. Cognitive and functional outcome after aneurysmal subarachnoid hemorrhage. Stroke 2010;41:e519–36.

64. Rosengart AJ, Schultheiss KE, Tolentino J, et al. Prognostic factors for outcome in patients with aneurysmal subarachnoid hemorrhage. Stroke 2007;38(8): 2315–21. Available at: http://www.ncbi.nlm.nih.gov/pubmed/17569871. Ac-cessed April 9, 2014.

65. Leung CH, Poon WS, Yu LM, et al. Apolipoprotein e Genotype and outcome in aneurysmal subarachnoid hemorrhage. Stroke 2002;33(2):548–52. Available at: http://stroke.ahajournals.org/cgi/doi/10.1161/hs0202.102326. Accessed April 22, 2014.

66. Claassen J, Hirsch L, Frontera J. Prognostic significance of continuous EEG monitoring in patients with poor-grade subarachnoid hemorrhage. Neurocrit Care 2006;4:103–12. Available at: http://link.springer.com/article/10.1385/NCC:4:2:103. Accessed April 23, 2014.

Intracranial Pressure Monitoring and Management of Intracranial Hypertension

Jon Perez-Barcena, MD, PhD[a],*,
Juan Antonio Llompart-Pou, MD, PhD[b], Kristine H. O'Phelan, MD[a]

KEYWORDS

- Intracranial pressure • Intracranial hypertension • Head injury

KEY POINTS

- Intracranial pressure is a reflection of the relationship between alterations in craniospinal volume and the ability of the craniospinal axis to accommodate the added volume.
- Intracranial pressure cannot be reliably estimated from any specific feature or CT finding and must be measured.
- Much information is available from ICP monitoring in addition to the measurement and display of absolute ICP.
- Elevated ICP is an important cause of secondary brain injury and is consistently associated with worse neurologic outcomes in patients with traumatic brain injury.
- ICP monitoring remains the cornerstone of management of patients with acute brain injury.

INTRODUCTION

The principles of intracranial pressure (ICP) were outlined by Monroe[1] and Kellie[2] in the 1820s. In essence, they noted that in adults, the brain is enclosed in a rigid case of bone and that the volume of its contents must remain constant if ICP is to remain constant. The intracranial compartment consists of approximately 83% brain, 11% cerebrospinal fluid (CSF), and 6% blood.

The relationship between ICP and intracranial volume is described by the pressure-volume curve that comprises 3 parts (**Fig. 1**). The first part of the curve is flat because compensatory reserves are adequate and ICP remains low despite increases in

Disclosures: None.
[a] Department of Neurology, University of Miami-Miller School of Medicine, 1120 Northwest 14th Street, Miami, FL 33136, USA; [b] Intensive Care Department, Son Espases Hospital, Crta Valldemossa 79, Palma de Mallorca, Balearic Islands 07010, Spain
* Corresponding author.
E-mail address: jperezbarcena@med.miami.edu

Crit Care Clin 30 (2014) 735–750
http://dx.doi.org/10.1016/j.ccc.2014.06.005
0749-0704/14/$ – see front matter © 2014 Elsevier Inc. All rights reserved.

criticalcare.theclinics.com

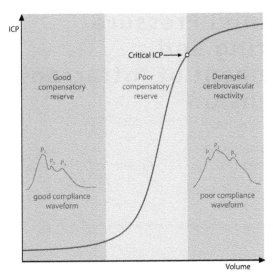

Fig. 1. Relationship between ICP and intracranial volume.

intracerebral volume. When these compensatory mechanisms become exhausted, the pressure-volume curve turns rapidly upwards in an exponential fashion. Intracranial compliance at this point is critically reduced and small increases in intracerebral volume cause a substantial increase in ICP. Thus, ICP is a reflection of the relationship between alterations in craniospinal volume and the ability of the craniospinal axis to accommodate the added volume.

Brain tissue pressure and ICP increase with each cardiac cycle; thus, the ICP waveform is a modified arterial pressure wave. The ICP pressure waveform has 3 distinct components that are related to physiologic parameters. The first peak (P1) is the percussive wave and reflects arterial pressure transmitted from the choroid plexus to the cerebral ventricle. The second peak (P2), often called the tidal wave, is thought due to brain tissue compliance. It is variable and generally increases in amplitude as compliance decreases; if it exceeds the level of the P1 waveform, it indicates a marked decrease in cerebral compliance. The P3 is due to the closure of the aortic valve and therefore illustrates the dicrotic notch (see **Fig. 1**).

METHODS OF ICP MONITORING

ICP cannot be reliably estimated from any specific clinical feature or CT finding and must be measured (**Fig. 2**). Different methods of monitoring ICP have been described but 2 methods are commonly used in clinical practice: intraventricular catheters and intraparenchymal catheter-tip microtransducer systems. The nondominant hemisphere is the preferred site for ICP monitor placement, unless the primary pathology affects the dominant hemisphere, in which case the dominant side is used.[3] Subarachnoid and epidural devices have much lower accuracy and are rarely used.[4,5] Measurement of lumbar CSF pressure does not provide a reliable estimate of ICP and may be dangerous in the presence of increased intracranial hypertension (ICH) because drainage of fluid from the lumbar space may result in a pressure gradient causing downward cerebral herniation.[6]

A ventricular catheter connected to an external strain gauge is the most accurate and low-cost method for ICP monitoring. The catheter is inserted into the lateral ventricle

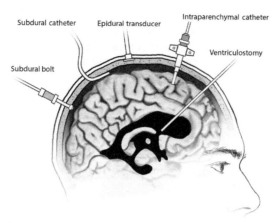

Fig. 2. Methods of monitoring ICP.

usually via a small right frontal bur hole. This method has proved reliable and to permit periodic rezeroing and it also allows the benefit of therapeutic CSF drainage.[7] The reference point for the transducer is the foramen of Monro, although in practical terms the external auditory meatus is often used. Some ventricular catheters have a pressure transducer within their lumen and the ICP waveform is generally of better quality than traditional fluid-filled catheters connected to an external transducer. Nevertheless, the potential risks of difficult positioning in the presence of ventricular compression and obstruction have led to alternative intracranial sites for ICP monitoring. Also, the use of intraventricular catheters is complicated by infection in 5% to 10% of cases.[8,9]

Microtransducer-tipped ICP monitors can be placed in the brain parenchyma through a twist drill craniostomy or a small bur hole or during a neurosurgical procedure requiring a craniotomy. ICP measurements obtained with intraparenchymal transducers correlate well with the values obtained with intraventricular catheters. Microtransducer systems are reliable and easy to use in the clinical setting. Recordings typically are stable over time with minor zero drift.[10] Their rates of infection or other complications are minimal.[11] A caveat to parenchymal monitoring, however, is that the measured pressure may not be representative of true CSF pressure because intraparenchymal pressure gradients may exist.[12] The cost of these devices is higher than the conventional ventricular system and does not allow therapeutic CSF drainage.

NORMAL AND PATHOLOGIC ICP

Normal ICP varies with age, body, position, and clinical conditions.[13] The normal ICP is 7 mm Hg to 15 mm Hg in a supine adult. The definition of ICH depends on the specific pathology and age, although ICP greater than 15 mm Hg is generally considered abnormal. Treatment is instituted at different levels, however, depending on the pathology. For example, ICP greater than 15 mm Hg may warrant treatment in a patient with hydrocephalus,[14] whereas after traumatic brain injury (TBI), treatment is indicated when ICP exceeds 20 mm Hg.[15]

The ICP threshold above which treatment should be initiated in TBI patients is still a matter of debate. The largest prospectively collected database study was published in 1991 by Marmarou and colleagues.[16] The investigators found a strong correlation between outcome and the number of hours with an ICP above 20 mm Hg. Similar results have been recently reported by Balestreri and colleagues[17] in a retrospective analysis performed on 492 TBI patients.

ICP is not evenly distributed in pathologic states because CSF does not circulate freely and intracranial CSF volume may be low because of brain swelling. In an injured brain, compartmentalization of pressures across the dura mater (falx cerebri or tentorium cerebelli) may create intraparenchymal pressure gradients between the supratentorial and infratentorial compartments. Bilateral monitoring has revealed differential pressures across the midline in the presence of hematomas and also in the absence of space-occupying lesions.[18,19] This relevant fact affects placement of the monitor typically to the side of injury. Important clinical patterns of ICP waves were described by Lundberg and colleagues in 1965.[20] They are as follows:

Lundberg waves (**Box 1**)

- A waves or plateau waves: have amplitudes of 50 mm Hg to 100 mm Hg, lasting 5 to 20 minutes. These waves are always associated with intracranial pathology. During such waves, it is common to observe evidence or early herniation, including bradycardia and hypertension. The etiology is uncertain, but it is postulated that as cerebral perfusion pressure (CPP) becomes inadequate to meet metabolic demand, cerebral vasodilation ensues and cerebral blood volume increases. This leads to a vicious circle, with further CPP decrease, predisposing patients to other plateau waves. If low CPP is not corrected, global cerebral ischemia ensues and eventually results in cerebrocirculatory arrest and brain death.
- B waves oscillate up to 50 mm Hg in amplitude with a frequency 0.5–2/min and are thought due to vasomotor center instability when CPP is unstable or at the lower limits of pressure autoregulation.
- C waves oscillate up to 20 mm Hg in amplitude and have a frequency of 4–8/min. These waves have been documented in healthy individuals and are thought to occur because of interaction between cardiac and respiratory cycles.

ICP: MORE THAN A NUMBER

An understanding of raised ICP encompasses an analysis of both intracranial volume and craniospinal compliance. Therefore, ICP is a reflection of the relationship between

---

Box 1
Information available from ICP monitoring

- ICP waveform: if P2 elevates or exceeds the level of the P1 waveform, there is a marked decrease in cerebral compliance.
- Lundberg A wave: amplitude of 50–100 mm Hg, lasting 5–20 minutes. The etiology is uncertain, but it is postulated that as CPP becomes inadequate to meet metabolic demand, cerebral vasodilation ensues and cerebral blood volume increases.
- Lundberg B wave: oscillate to 50 mm Hg in amplitude with a frequency 0.5–2/min. It is thought due to vasomotor center instability.
- Lundberg C wave: oscillating and up to 20 mm Hg in amplitude and has a frequency of 4–8/min. It is thought to occur because of interaction between cardiac and respiratory cycles.
- CPP: difference between mean arterial BP and ICP. It reflects cerebral blood flow.
- PRx: index to describe cerebrovascular pressure reactivity. It is derived from continuous monitoring and analysis of slow waves in arterial BP and ICP.
- RAP: index to describe the compensatory reserve of the brain. It is the relationship between the amplitude of the ICP waveform and the mean ICP over 1–3 minutes.

alterations in craniospinal volume and the ability of the craniospinal axis to accommodate added volume.

Much information is available from ICP monitoring in addition to the measurement and display of absolute ICP. CPP is easily calculated as the difference between mean arterial pressure (MAP) and ICP and is a measure of the pressure gradient across the cerebral vascular bed. Pathologic ICP waveforms can be identified obtaining cerebrovascular pressure reactivity and pressure volume compensatory reserve.

The ICP response to slow spontaneous changes in blood pressure (BP) depends on the pressure-reactivity of cerebral vessels. A pressure reactivity index (PRx) can be derived from a continuous monitoring and analysis of slow waves in arterial BP and ICP.[21] PRx is the linear correlation coefficient between MAP and ICP and its value ranges from −1 to +1. When the cerebrovascular bed is normally reactive, an increase in BP leads to cerebral vasoconstriction within 5 to 15 seconds and a secondary reduction in cerebral blood volume and ICP. Opposite effects occur when MAP is reduced.

When the cerebrovascular reactivity is impaired, changes in BP passively transmit to the cerebral blood volume and ICP. PRx is determined by calculating the correlation coefficient or consecutive time averaged data points of ICP and MAP recorded over a 4-minute period. A negative value for PRx results when BP is inversely correlated with ICP. This indicates normal cerebrovasular reactivity, whereas a positive value suggests a nonreactive cerebral circulation. PRx correlates with standard measures of cerebral autor-regulation based on transcranial Doppler ultrasonography and abnormal values are predictive of poor outcome after TBI.[4] PRx can be monitored continuously and has been used to define individual CPP targets after TBI.[22]

The relation between ICP and changes in intracerebral volume can be used to define an index of compensatory reserve (RAP) (see **Box 1**). RAP is the relationship between BP and the mean ICP over 1 to 3 minutes.[23] Values of this index also range from −1 to +1. The first segment of the ICP-volume curve is flat, reflecting a lack of synchronization between BP and ICP and representing good compensatory reserve. Here the RAP is zero and the ICP waveform amplitude is low. On the steep part of the curve, when compensatory reserves begin to fail, BP varies directly with ICP and RAP is +1. ICP waveform amplitude begins to increase as mean ICP increases, at first slowly and then more rapidly as compensatory reserves are exhausted. Finally, on the terminal part of the curve, derangement of the cerebral vasculature and a decrease in pulse pressure transmission from the arterial bed to the intracranial compartment results in low or absent ICP waveform amplitude. RAP, therefore, can be used to indicate a patient's position on the pressure-volume curve and may be used to predict the response to treatment and the risk of clinical deterioration or herniation. RAP less than 0.5 in association with ICP greater than 20 mm Hg is predictive or poor outcome after TBI.[23]

CONTROVERSIES OF ICP MONITORING

Elevated ICP is an important cause of secondary brain injury and is consistently associated with worse neurologic outcomes in patients after TBI.[24,25] Given this, ICP monitoring is currently a level II recommendation from the Brain Trauma Foundation in patients with severe TBI Glasgow Coma Scale less than or equal to 8 derived from nonrandomized controlled trials.[26] Despite guidelines that support the role of ICP monitoring in the management of severe TBI, there still exist significant variations in practice, and patients sometimes undergo ICP lowering therapy without ICP monitors.[27,28]

Previous studies were observational and nonrandomized; therefore, the decision to insert an ICP monitor was already made by a clinical team prior to enrollment. This creates significant selection bias in these studies. For example, the decision to place an ICP monitor may be influenced by factors relating to a patient's premorbid conditions, the severity of the current TBI, and center-specific practices and preferences. Consequently, even with multivariable adjustment, determining an unbiased outcome estimate for ICP monitors in these studies is extremely difficult. This is exacerbated by the generally small samples sizes of the published studies that limit adequate statistical adjustment.

Although selection bias explains the mixed results that were found, ICP monitoring may still influence outcomes independently and, therefore, deserves closer attention. A distinction must be made between the information obtained from the ICP monitor and the interventions instituted based on this information. For example, change in management based on ICP measurements can be instituted using an ICP goal, a CPP goal, or a less used, volume-targeted strategy (ie, Lund protocol). The principles of the Lund protocol include the prevention of brain edema formation by reducing fluid shift from capillaries into brain parenchymal by preserving capillary colloid osmotic pressure with blood products, albumin, and diuretics and reduction of capillary hydrostatic pressure (CPP 50–70 mm Hg) with the α_2-agonist, clonidine; β-blockade with metoprolol; low-dose thiopental; and dihydroegotamine. Vasoactive medications, such as dobutamine and norepinephrine, are avoided with the goal of improving cerebral microcirculation. Ideal ICP and CPP target values have yet to be identified. Furthermore, clinicians may decide to use only the quantitative value of ICP whereas others may additionally use the ICP waveform to direct management.[14]

Ideally, the information gained from these monitoring devices will lead to interventions that improve outcomes. Yet, many current therapies for increased ICP, such as sedation and pharmacologic paralysis, are potentially associated with adverse effects and worse outcomes in critically ill patients. In order for any monitoring device to independently improve outcome, it must (1) be used in the appropriate patient population, (2) be accurate and reliable, (3) have minimal complications, (4) be correctly interpreted within the clinical context, (5) be acted on in a standardized and reproducible manner, and (6) dictate interventions that generate positive outcomes. By definition, a monitoring technique is not a therapeutic intervention and without interventions the natural course of an illness cannot be modified. Consequently, to provide benefit for monitoring, appropriate therapy should derive from the information acquired by the monitoring itself.

Recently, the Benchmark Evidence from South American Trials: Treatment of Intracranial Pressure[29] was published. This trial was a prospective, randomized, outcome-masked clinical trial led by researchers at the University of Washington that randomized 324 patients of 13 years of age or older with severe TBI presenting within 24 hours of injury from several centers in Bolivia and Ecuador to either TBI management based on ICP monitoring or TBI management conducted according to a protocol based exclusively on serial imaging CT scans and clinical examination. The primary outcome was a composite of survival time, duration, and level of impaired consciousness, functional status at 3 and 6 months, and cognitive status at 6 months as analyzed through several batteries of neuropsychological tests. The overall composite outcome for each patient was calculated as the average of the percentiles from the 21 measures, displayed on a scale from 0 to 100, with lower percentiles representing worse outcome. The final analysis of this 5-year study demonstrated no statistical difference between the 2 groups (composite score 56 in the pressure monitoring group vs 53 in the imaging clinical examination group; $P = .49$). Six-month mortality also was not significantly different between the 2 groups (39% in the pressure-monitoring group vs 41% in the nonimaging clinical examination group; $P = .6$). Neither was the median length of stay in the ICU (12 days in the pressure monitoring group vs 9 days in the imaging clinical examination group; $P = .25$), although the number of days during which brain-specific treatments were performed (eg, administration of hyperosmolar fluids and use of hyperventilation) throughout the ICU stay was significantly higher in the imaging-guided group than in the pressure monitoring group (4.8 days vs 3.4 days; $P = .002$). The distribution of serious adverse events was also similar in both groups.

A limitation of the study is that the trial was not sufficiently powered to detect a mortality difference between both groups. In addition, differences in injury characteristics, prehospital, ICU, and post-ICU processes of care and the observation of delayed mortality due to medical complications, which accounts for more than one-third of deaths subsequent to TBI in Latin America, may render questionable any extrapolation of epidemiologic or treatments studies from the developing to developed world.

To manage patients with severe TBI based solely on clinical and serial imaging examinations implies keeping patients with severe neurologic injuries without proper sedation (or submitting them to repeated wake-up tests for clinical examination). This strategy that has been shown to have variable effects on ICP, brain metabolism, and brain tissue oxygenation.[30,31]

As the investigators point out, their study does not question the importance of ICP. To the contrary, the result suggests that patients in the imaging-guided group were treated more aggressively for ICH than patients in the ICP group. The main difference was the way ICP was measured or inferred either by direct monitoring in the ICP-directed group or indirectly by imaging studies and clinical examination in the imaging-guided group. One considerable limitation of this study is the lack of ICP data in the control group. This study should not change the current practice of ICP monitoring in patients who are at high risk of ICH. It supports aggressive treatment of ICH.[32]

Without ICP monitoring, considerable information is missing and objective management of the patient is not achievable. Currently, therapeutic strategies are oriented to reduce raised ICP. Moreover, ICP monitors are cost effective and have an acceptably low complication rate. They offer a high yield of information gained and should be the cornerstone of all critical care management of acute brain injury.[33]

MANAGEMENT OF ICH

Aggressive treatment of ICH is effective in reducing mortality and improving outcome.[34,35] Because of potential side effects of therapy and intensive ICP monitoring, identifying patients at risk for developing ICH is crucial in preventing pathologic changes that may result in poor outcome and increased mortality.

After trauma, the injured brain is characterized by huge pathophysiologic heterogeneity: ischemic areas (cytotoxic edema) coexist with areas with blood-brain barrier disruptions (vasogenic edema), contusions, and normal brain parenchyma. The proportion of each of these areas likely depends on the severity of the TBI. Increased ICP can be related to intracranial mass lesions, contusional injuries, vascular engorgement, and brain edema. The management of ICH revolves around reduction in volume of 1 of the 3 intracranial compartments: brain, blood, and CSF.[36]

General Measures

Meticulous multidisciplinary management of critically ill patients is paramount to the success of any ICU (**Box 2**).[37] The airway should be secured early and immediately.

Box 2
Management of ICH

A. General management

- Head of bed at 30°C
- Temperature below 38°C
- Glucose control: keep blood glucose between 80 and 160 mg/dL
- Serum Na between 145 and 155 mmol/L; serum osmolality less than 320 mOsm/kg
- Hemoglobin level above 8–9 g/dL
- Oxygen saturation above 96% and Pao_2 between 80 mm Hg and 120 mm Hg
- Normoventilation: $Paco_2$ between 35 mm Hg and 40 mm Hg
- Normovolemia: CVP 7–11 mm Hg
- Normotension: MAP greater than 80 mm Hg or CPP greater than 60 mm Hg
- Analgesia/sedation

B. First-tier measures

- CSF drainage
- Osmotherapy: mannitol 0.5–2 g/kg bolus as needed for ICP greater than 20 mm Hg
  3% hypertonic saline; 250-mL bolus as needed for ICP greater than 20 mm Hg
- Increased sedation
- Paralytic agent

C. Second-tier measures

- Moderate hypothermia
- Decompressive craniectomy
- Barbiturate coma

Once the airway has been secured, ventilator settings should be adjusted to the optimal setting required to maintain an O_2 saturation above 90%, a Pao_2 between 80 mm Hg and 120 mm Hg, and a $Paco_2$ within the 35 mm Hg to 40 mm Hg range.[38,39] The mode of ventilation should be selected based on patient response and comfort. Prophylactic hyperventilation is discouraged based on studies showing tissue ischemia below a $Paco_2$ of 25 mm Hg.[38]

Maintenance of euvolemia is important for hemodynamic stability. Central venous pressure (CVP) goals are 8 mm Hg to 12 mm Hg or pulmonary capillary wedge pressure of 10 mm Hg to 15 mm Hg. Normal saline is the preferred solution for fluid bolus/maintenance in the neurocritical care unit.[40,41] Prophylactic use of osmotic agents is not advocated due to their volume-depleting effect and questionable benefit.[42] Avoidance of hypotension is paramount in early management of acute brain injury because the recently injured brain is particularly susceptible to ischemic secondary injury. Systolic BP must be kept above 90 mm Hg.[39] Guidelines recognize the inconsistent relationship between systolic and MAP and that it may be valuable to maintain a MAP considerably above those represented by a SBP greater than 90 mm Hg, but there are currently no data to support this. When ICP monitoring is available, MAPs should be maintained to keep CPP between 50 mm Hg and 70 mm Hg[43] but typically greater than 60 mm Hg. Norepinephrine is the vasopressor of choice due to its favorable hemodynamic effects; however, it may cause reflex bradycardia.[44,45] Besides normal saline, the use of albumin (5%) 250 mL intravenous (IV) bolus to achieve the CVP goal may augment volume expansion.

Strict glucose control is essential to the management of acutely injured brain, because hyperglycemia has been correlated with poor outcome.[46,47] Intensive insulin therapy to keep the blood glucose level between 80 and 110 mg/dL is shown to improve outcome and reduce mortality in medical and surgical ICUs.[48,49] Several experimental[50] and clinical studies[51] have shown, however, that intensive systemic glucose lowering reduces brain glucose concentration, a risk factor for poor outcome. Currently, a less-aggressive glucose target of 80 to 140 mg/dL is suggested for patients with acute brain injury.

Maintenance of normothermia at 36°C to 37°C augments ICP management and may be done using antipyretics and cooling blankets,[52] surface cooling, or intravascular devices.

The use of sedation and analgesia is an important management strategy, especially in patients with ICH. Propofol is the preferred agent for short-term sedation due to its short half-life, making frequent clinical examinations possible. It also has a favorable effect on cerebral hemodynamics, reducing ICP.[53] A ceiling dose of 5 mg/kg/h is advocated to prevent complications related to propofol infusion syndrome. Fentanyl infusion may also be used to provide analgesia. Also, short-acting benzodiazepines, such as lorazepam and midazolam, may be used.[54] Lorazepam requires a propylene glycol diluent, however, and high-dose infusions of lorazepam are avoided due risk for propylene glycol toxicity.

Head-of-bed elevation to 30° has been shown to reduce ICP while maintaining an adequate CPP in brain-injured patients. Maintenance of straight head position prevents kinking of the jugular venous system and facilitates venous drainage.[55,56]

A significant number of patients with acute brain injury are at risk for early seizures. Seizures acutely increase the ICP and amplify metabolic demand. Because of this, patients should be given seizure prophylaxis with an anticonvulsant for 7 days postinjury. Fosphenytoin (loading dose of 20 mg/kg IV over 1 hour and maintenance of 100 mg every 8 hours daily) or levetiracetam (1000 mg every12 hours daily) may be used.[57–59]

Nutrition is an important part of management of acute brain injury patients. When started within 72 hours after injury, nutrition may decrease infection and other complications. Patients with TBI should be given 140% resting metabolic expenditure with 15% protein.[60] It is recommended that patients be fed to attain this full caloric intake by day 7 after injury.

CSF Drainage

Drainage of CSF is frequently used in the management of ICH. This therapy is simple and cost effective and overrides the often serious systemic complications related to pharmacologic therapy.[61]

Osmotherapy

Two osmotic agents are currently in use in most neurocritical care units: mannitol and hypertonic saline. Both are highly effective in reducing acutely elevated ICP in various clinical conditions, with almost immediate effect lasting for several hours. Mannitol has several mechanisms of action. An immediate effect from bolus administration results from plasma expansion with reduction of blood viscosity, improvement in microvascular cerebral blood flow, cerebral oxygenation, and CPP with reduction in cerebral blood volume due to autoregulatory vasoconstriction and ultimately lowering of ICP. A slightly delayed effect, occurring within 15 to 30 minutes and lasting for up to 6 hours, results from a direct osmotic effect on neural cells with reduction in total brain water.[62–64]

Hypertonic saline use in neurocritical care is increasing due to its favorable effect on systemic hemodynamics, ease of use, and proved efficacy. Several preparations have been studied clinically, ranging from 1.5% to 30%. Hypertonic saline has similar efficacy with mannitol and may be used interchangeably, especially in patients with a high osmolar gap.[65–67]

Decompressive Craniectomy

In the past decade, there has been an ongoing debate about the role of secondary decompressive craniectomy in the management of high ICP. A Cochrane systematic review updated in 2008 concluded that there was no evidence to support the routine use of decompressive craniectomy to reduce unfavorable outcomes in adults with TBI and refractory high ICP. The same review concluded, however, that decompressive craniectomy could be an option in the pediatric population when maximal medical treatment fails to control ICP. This recommendation was based on a single randomized controlled trial (RCT) published by Taylor and colleagues.[68,69]

Decompressive Craniectomy in Patients with Severe Traumatic Brain Injury (DECRA) was a multicenter RCT conducted in 15 hospitals in Australia, New Zealand, and Saudi Arabia designed to test the efficacy of bifrontotemporoparietal decompressive craniectomy in adults aged below 60 years with a severe TBI in whom first-tier therapeutic measures failed to control high ICP to below 20 mm Hg.[70] Refractory high ICP was defined in this study as "a spontaneous (not stimulated) increase in ICP for more than 15 min (continuously or intermittently) within a 1-h period, despite optimized first-tier interventions." First-tier therapies were defined according to the Brain Trauma Foundation guidelines.

In the DECRA study, 3478 patients were assessed for eligibility and only 155 were enrolled (4.5%). Seventy-three patients were randomized to decompressive craniectomy and 82 were assigned to standard care. The baseline characteristics of the 2 groups were well balanced with the unlucky exception of the number of patients with bilateral unreactive pupils, which was significantly higher in the decompressive craniectomy group (27%) than in the control group (12%). Median ICP during 12 hours before randomization was 20 mm Hg in both arms. After randomization, mean ICP was significantly lower in the decompressive craniectomy group (14.4 mm Hg vs 19.1 mm Hg; P<.001). Despite the significant reduction in the duration of mechanical ventilation and days in the ICU, decompressive craniectomy increased the likelihood of a poor outcome. Unfavorable outcomes occurred in 51 patients (70%) in the decompressive craniectomy group and in 42 patients (51%) in the control group. These differences in outcome vanished, however, after adjusting the results for the pupillary reactivity covariate. After adjustment, there were no statistically significant differences in the dichotomized 6-month outcome. The investigators' main conclusion was that decompressive craniectomy decreased ICP and the length of stay in the ICU but was associated with more unfavorable outcomes.

Despite the negative findings of DECRA, the global claim that decompressive craniectomy increases unfavorable outcome may be overstated. Specifically, DECRA does not address unilateral decompressive craniectomy in patients with refractory ICP and focal brain injury. It is premature to change clinical practice based on a single study and decompressive craniectomy should not be disregarded in certain patients with high ICP refractory to first-line therapeutic measures. Given the dismal prognosis without further intervention in these patients, it is reasonable to include this technique as a last resort in any type of protocol-driven management when conventional therapeutic measures have failed, the presence of operable masses has been ruled out, and the patient may still have a chance of a functional outcome.[71]

Barbiturate Coma

In patients with preserved flow-metabolism coupling, barbiturate-induced cerebral metabolic suppression is an effective way of reducing ICP refractory to osmotherapy. Barbiturates reduce cerebral metabolism with concomitant reduction in cerebral blood flow, thereby decreasing ICP. In addition, barbiturates have neuroprotective properties, including free radical scavenger function, apoptosis inhibition, and reduction in intracerebral pyruvate and lactate production.[72,73]

A minimum barbiturate dose required to control ICP is advocated with frequent dose adjustments. There have been no consistent predictable relationships between cerebral metabolism and barbiturate levels, precluding the clinical use of drug levels. Continuous electroencephalographic (EEG) monitoring is recommended to prevent overdosing as the maximum effect on metabolic suppression, cerebral blood flow, and ICP reduction is achieved with an EEG pattern showing 1 to 2 bursts per minute.[74] Overdosing is exhibited by an isoelectric EEG pattern, at which point further bolus dosing or increases in the infusion rate results in complications from side effects rather than beneficial effects on ICP control.

Despite its efficacy, barbiturate therapy has a variable effect on outcome and no benefit has been shown with prophylactic administration. Complications include systemic hypotension that almost always occurs with barbiturate therapy. Other side effects of barbiturate coma include immune suppression and sepsis, electrolyte abnormalities, ileus, and hepatic and renal dysfunction. Because of significant potential adverse effects with no clear effect on long-term outcome, high-dose barbiturate therapy is considered a second-tier treatment strategy for ICH intractable to osmotic agents.[75]

Hypothermia

Induced hypothermia is effective in reducing ICP by suppressing all cerebral metabolic activities, thereby reducing CBF. It has been found cytoprotective in animal models, reducing ischemia-induced release of glutamate. The use of hypothermia for patients at high risk for high ICP has shown variable results.[76,77] The increased amount of resources associated with its use, the difficulty in consistently delivering therapeutic hypothermia protocols across different institutions, and potential infectious adverse effects make hypothermia a second-tier therapy in refractory ICP.[77,78]

A significant number of issues remain unresolved with respect to therapeutic temperature modulation to treat patients with brain injury. These include the ideal target temperature, patient selection, mode of administration of cooling, timing of intervention, duration of treatment, and duration and rapidity of rewarming.[79] Many of this ambiguity applies, however, to the use of therapeutic hypothermia as an initial neuroprotective therapy used immediately after injury rather than a strategy for treating elevated ICP. Most data support that this technique is consistently effective when used to treat ICP.

SUMMARY

In summary, ICP monitoring remains a cornerstone of management of patients with acute brain injury. A landmark study offering equipoise as to whether ICP management makes a difference shows that an ICP-based management was more efficient by shortening ICU length of stay and decreasing the number of interventions to achieve the same outcome. Methods of evaluating the loss of cerebral autoregulation and the compliance and compensatory reserve of the brain may offer future tools to further refine the optimal management in care of these patients.

REFERENCES

1. Monro A. Observations on the structure and function of the nervous system. Edinburgh: Creech & Johnson; 1823. p. 5.
2. Kellie G. An account of the appearances observed in the dissection of two of the three individuals presumed to have perished in the storm of the 3rd, and whose bodies were discovered in the vicinity of Leith on the morning of the 4th November 1821 with some reflections on the pathology of the brain. Trans Med Chir Sci, Edinburgh 1824;1:84–169.
3. Lavinio A, Menon D. Intracranial pressure: why we monitor it, how to monitor it, what to do with the number and what's the future? Curr Opin Anaesthesiol 2011; 24:117–23.
4. Brain Trauma Foundation, American Association of Neurological Surgeons, Congress of Neurological Surgeons, Joint Section on Neurotrauma and Critical Care. Guidelines for the management of severe traumatic brain injury. VII. Intracranial pressure monitoring technology. J Neurotrauma 2007;24: S45–54.
5. Citerio G, Andrews PJ. Intracranial pressure. Part two: clinical applications and technology. Intensive Care Med 2004;30:1882–5.
6. Steiner LA, Andrews PJ. Monitoring the injured brain: ICP and CBF. Br J Anaesth 2006;97:26–38.
7. Zhong J, Dujovny M, Park HK, et al. Advances in ICP monitoring techniques. Neurol Res 2003;25:339–50.
8. Lozier AP, Sciaca RR, Romagnoli MF, et al. Ventriculostomy-related infections: a criticial review of the literatura. Neurosurgery 2002;51:170–81.
9. Mayhall CG, Archer NH, Lamb VA, et al. Ventriculostomy-related infections. A prospective epidemiologic study. N Engl J Med 1984;310:553–9.
10. Koskinen LO, Olivecrona M. Clinical experience with the intraparenchymal intracranial pressure monitoring Codman Microsensor system. Neurosurgery 2005; 56:693–8.
11. Martinez-Manas RM, Santamarta D, de Campos JM, et al. Camino intracranial pressure monitor: prospective study of accuracy and complications. J Neurol Neurosurg Psychiatry 2000;69:82–6.
12. Sahuquillo J, Poca MA, Arribas M, et al. Interhemispheric supratentorial intracranial pressure gradients in head-injured patients: are they clinically important? J Neurosurg 1999;90:16–26.
13. Albeck MJ, Skak C, Nielsen PR, et al. Age dependency of resistance to cerebrospinal fluid outflow. J Neurosurg 1998;89:275–8.
14. Czosnyka M, Pickard JD. Monitoring and interpretation of intracranial pressure. J Neurol Neurosurg Psychiatry 2004;75:813–21.
15. Brain Trauma Foundation, American Associatin of Neurological Surgeons, Congress of Neurological Surgeons, Joint Section on Neurotrauma and Critical Care. Guidelines for the management of severe traumatic brain injury. VIII. Intracranial pressure thresholds. J Neurotrauma 2007;24:S55–8.
16. Marmarou A, Anderson RL, Ward JD, et al. Impact of ICP instability and hypotension on outcome in patients with severe head trauma. J Neurosurg 1991;75:S59–66.

17. Balestreri M, Czosnyka M, Hutchinson P, et al. Impact of intracranial pressure and cerebral perfusion pressure on severe disability and mortality after head injury. Neurocritical Care 2006;4:8–13.

18. Wolfla CE, Luerssen TG, Bowman RM. Regional brain tissue pressure gradients created by expanding extradural temporal mass lesion. J Neurosurg 1997;86: 506–10.

19. Mindermann T, Gratzl O. Interhemispheric pressure gradients in severe head trauma in humans. Acta Neurochir Suppl 1998;71:56–8.

20. Lundberg N, Troupp J, Lorin H. Continous recording of the ventricular fluid pressure in patients with severe acute traumatic brain injury. A preliminary report. J Neurosurg 1965;22:581–90.

21. Czosnyka M, Smielewski P, Kirkpatrick P, et al. Continous assessment of the cerebral vasomotor reactivity in head injury. Neurosurgery 1997;41:11–7.

22. Steiner LA, Czosnyka M, Piechnik SK, et al. Continous monitoring of cerebrovascular pressure reactivity allows determination of optimal cerebral perfusion pressure in patients with traumatic brain injury. Crit Care Med 2002;30:733–8.

23. Czosnyka M, Guazzo E, Whitehouse M, et al. Significance of intracranial pressure waveform analysis after head injury. Acta Neurochir (Wien) 1996;138:531–41.

24. Saul TG, Ducker TB. Effect of intracranial pressure monitoring and aggressive treatment on mortality in severe head injury. J Neurosurg 1982;56:498–503.

25. Juul N, Morris GF, Marshall SB, et al. Intracranial hypertension and cerebral perfusion pressure: influence on neurological deterioration and outcome in severe head injury. The Executive Committee of the International Selfotel Trial. J Neurosurg 2000;92:1–6.

26. Brain Trauma Foundation, American Associatin of Neurological Surgeons, Congress of Neurological Surgeons, Joint Section on Neurotrauma and Critical Care. Guidelines for the management of severe traumatic brain injury. VI. Indications for intracranial pressure monitoring. J Neurotrauma 2007;24: S37–44.

27. Bulger EM, Nathens AB, Rivara FP, et al. Management of severe head injury: institutional variations in care and effect on outcome. Crit Care Med 2002;30: 1870–6.

28. Lane PL, Skoretz TG, Doig G, et al. Intracranial pressure monitoring and outcomes after traumatic brain injury. Can J Surg 2000;43:442–8.

29. Chesnut RM, Temkin N, Carney N, et al. A trial of intracranial pressure monitoring in traumatic brain injury. N Engl J Med 2012;367:2471–81.

30. Helbok R, Kurtz P, Schmidt MJ, et al. Effects of the neurological wake-up test on clinical examination, intracranial pressure, brain metabolism and brain tissue oxygenation in severely brain injured patients. Crit Care 2012;16:R226.

31. Skoglund K, Hillared L, Purins K, et al. The neurologic wake up test does not alter cerebral energy metabolism and oxygenation in patients with severe traumatic brain injury. Neurocrit Care 2014;20:413–26.

32. Hartl R, Stieg PE. Intracranial pressure is still number 1 despite BEST: TRIP study. World Neurosurg 2013;79:598–604.

33. Oddo M, Villa F, Citerio G. Brain multimodality monitoring: an update. Curr Opin Crit Care 2012;18:111–8.

34. Becker DP, Miller JD, Ward JD, et al. The outcome from severe head injury with early diagnosis and intensive management. J Neurosurg 1977;47:491–502.

35. Qureshi AI, Geocadin RG, Suarez JI, et al. Long-term outcome after medical reversal of transtentorial herniation in patients with supratentorial mass lesions. Crit Care Med 2000;28:1556–64.

36. Lescot T, Abdennour L, Boch AL, et al. Treatment of intracranial hypertension. Curr Opin Crit Care 2008;14:129–34.

37. Latorre JG, Greer DM. Management of acute intracranial hypertension. Neurologist 2009;15:193–207.

38. Brain Trauma Foundation, American Association of Neurological Surgeons, Congress of Neurological Surgeons, Joint Section on Neurotrauma and Critical Care. Guidelines for the management of severe traumatic brain injury. XIV. Hyperventilation. J Neurotrauma 2007;24:S87–90.

39. Brain Trauma Foundation, American Association of Neurological Surgeons, Congress of Neurological Surgeons, Joint Section on Neurotrauma and Critical Care. Guidelines for the management of severe traumatic brain injury. I. Blood pressure and oxygenation. J Neurotrauma 2007;24:S7–13.

40. Choi PT, Yip G, Quinonez LG, et al. Crystalloids vs colloids in fluid resuscitation: a systematic review. Crit Care Med 1999;27:200–10.

41. Zornow MH, Prough DS. Fluid management in patients with traumatic brain injury. New Horiz 1995;3:488–98.

42. Brain Trauma Foundation, American Association of Neurological Surgeons, Congress of Neurological Surgeons, Joint Section on Neurotrauma and Critical Care. Guidelines for the management of severe traumatic brain injury. II. Hyperosmolar therapy. J Neurotrauma 2007;24:S14–20.

43. Brain Trauma Foundation, American Association of Neurological Surgeons, Congress of Neurological Surgeons, Joint Section on Neurotrauma and Critical Care. Guidelines for the management of severe traumatic brain injury. IX. Cerebral Perfusion Thresholds. J Neurotrauma 2007;24:S59–64.

44. Johnston AJ, Steiner LA, Chatfield DA, et al. Effect of cerebral perfusion pressure augmentation with dopamine and norepinephrine on global and focal brain oxygenation after traumatic brain injury. Intensive Care Med 2004;30: 791–7.

45. Steiner LA, Johnston AJ, Czosnyka M, et al. Direct comparision of cerebrovascular effects of norepinephrine and dopamine in head-injured patients. Crit Care Med 2004;32:1049–54.

46. Whitcomb BW, Pradhan EK, Pittas AG, et al. Impact of admission hyperglycemia on hospital mortality in various intensive care unit populations. Crit Care Med 2005;33:2772–7.

47. Frontera JA, Fernandez A, Claassen J, et al. Hyperglycemia after SAH: predictors, associated complications and impact on outcome. Stroke 2006;37:199–203.

48. Van den Berghe G, Wilmer AG, Hermans G, et al. Intensive insulin therapy in the medical ICU. N Engl J Med 2006;354:449–61.

49. Van den Berghe G, Wouters P, Weekers F, et al. Intensive insulin therapy in the critically ill patients. N Engl J Med 2001;345:1359–67.

50. Hopwood SE, Parkin MC, Bezzima EL, et al. Transient changes in cortical glucose and lactate levels associated with peri infarct depolarisations, studied with rapid sampling microdialysis. J Cereb Blood Flow Metab 2005;25: 391–401.

51. Vespa P, Booyaputthikul R, McArthur DL, et al. Intensive insulin therapy reduces microdialysis glucose values without altering glucose utilization or improving the lactate/pyruvate ratio after traumatic brain injury. Crit Care Med 2006;34:850–6.

52. Tokutomi T, Morimoto K, Miyagi T, et al. Optimal temperaturye for the management of severe traumatic brain injury: effect of hypothermia on intracranial pressure, systemic and intracranial hemodynamics, and metabolism. Neurosurgery 2003;52:102–11.

53. Kelly DF, Goodale DB, Williams J, et al. Propofol in the treatment of moderate and severe head injury: a randomized, prospective double blinded pilot trial. J Neurosurg 1999;90:1042–52.
54. Jacobi J, Fraser GL, Coursin DB, et al. Clinical practice guidelines for the sustained use of sedatives and analgesics in the critically ill adult. Crit Care Med 2002;30:119–41.
55. Ng I, Lim J, Wong HB. Effects of head posture on pressure, and cerebral oxygenation. Neurosurgery 2004;54:593–7.
56. Feldman Z, Kanter MJ, Robertson CS, et al. Effect of head elevation on intracranial pressure, cerebral perfusion pressure, and cerebral blood flow in head injured patients. J Neurosurg 1992;76:207–11.
57. Temkin NR, Dikmen SS, Wilensky AJ, et al. A randomized, double-blind study of phenytoin for the prevention of post traumatic seizures. N Engl J Med 1990;323: 497–502.
58. Brain Trauma Foundation, American Association of Neurological Surgeons, Congress of Neurological Surgeons, Joint Section on Neurotrauma and Critical Care. Guidelines for the management of severe traumatic brain injury. XIII. Antiseizure prophyaxis. J Neurotrauma 2007;24:S83–6.
59. Inaba K, Menaker J, Branco BC, et al. A prospective multicenter comparison of levetiracetam versus phenytoin for early posttraumatic seizure prophylaxis. J Trauma Acute Care Surg 2013;74(3):766–71 [discussion: 771–3].
60. Brain Trauma Foundation, American Association of Neurological Surgeons, Congress of Neurological Surgeons, Joint Section on Neurotrauma and Critical Care. Guidelines for the management of severe traumatic brain injury. XII. Nutrition. J Neurotrauma 2007;24:S77–82.
61. Kerr ME, Weber BB, Sereika SM, et al. Dose response to cerebrospinal fluid drainage on cerebral perfusion in traumatic brain injured adults. Neurosurg Focus 2001;11:E1.
62. Cruz J, Miner ME, Allen SJ, et al. Continuous monitoring of cerebral oxygenation in acute brain injury: injection of manitol during hyperventilation. J Neurosurg 1990;73:725–30.
63. Muizelaar JP, Wei EP, Kontos HA, et al. Mannitol causes compensatory cerebral vasoconstriction and vasodilation in response to blood viscosity changes. J Neurosurg 1983;59:822–8.
64. Donato T, Shapira Y, Artru A, et al. Effect of mannitol on cerebrospinal fluid dynamics and brain tissue edema. Anesth Analg 1994;78:58–66.
65. Munar F, Ferrer AM, de Nadal M, et al. Cerebral hemodynamics effects of 7.2% hypertonic saline in patients with head injury and raised intracranial pressure. N Neurotrauma 2000;17:41–51.
66. Suarez JI. Hypertonic saline for cerebral edema and elevated intracranial pressure. Cleve Clin J Med 2004;71(Suppl 1):S9–13.
67. Qureshi AI, Suarez JI. Use of hypertonic saline solutions in treatment of cerebral edema and intracranial hypertension. Crit Care Med 2000;28:3301–13.
68. Sahuquillo J, Arikan F. Decompressive craniectomy for the treatement of refractory high intracranial pressure in traumatic brain injury. Cochrane Database Syst Rev 2006;(1):CD003983.
69. Taylor A, Butt W, Rosenfeld J, et al. A randomized trial of very early decompressive craniectomy in children with traumatic brain injury and sustained intracranial hypertension. Childs Nerv Syst 2001;17:154–62.
70. Cooper DJ, Rosenfeld JV, Murray L, et al. Decompressive craniectomy in diffuse traumatic brain injury. N Engl J Med 2011;364:1493–502.

71. Hutchinson PJ, Menon DK, Kirkpatrick JP. Decompressive craniectomy in traumatic brain injury? Time for randomized trials? Acta Neurochir 2004; 1147:1–3.
72. Cormio M, Gopinath SP, Valadka A, et al. Cerebral hemodynamics effects of pentobarbital coma in head injured patients. J Neurotrauma 1999;16:927–36.
73. Lee MW, Deppe SA, Sipperly ME, et al. The efficacy of barbiturate coma in the management of uncontrolled intracranial hypertension following neurosurgical trauma. J Neurotrauma 1994;11:325–31.
74. Warner DS, Taraoka S, Wu B, et al. Elecroencephalographic burst suppression is not required to elicit maximal neuroprotection from pentobarbital in a rat model of focal cerebral ischemia. Anesthesiology 1996;84:1475–84.
75. Brain Trauma Foundation, American Association of Neurological Surgeons, Congress of Neurological Surgeons, Joint Section on Neurotrauma and Critical Care. Guidelines for the management of severe traumatic brain injury. XI. Anesthetics, analgesics and sedatives. J Neurotrauma 2007;24:S71–6.
76. Clifton GL, Miller ER, Choi SC, et al. Lack of effect of induction of hypothermia after acute brain injury. N Engl J Med 2001;344:556–63.
77. Polderman KH, Tjon Tjin Joe R, Peederman SM, et al. Effects of therapeutic hypothermia on intracranial pressure and outcome in patients with severe head injury. Intensive Care Med 2002;28:1563–73.
78. Sahuquillo J, Perez Barcena J, Biestro A, et al. Intravascular cooling for rapid induction of moderate hypothermia in severely head injured patients: results of a multicenter study (Intracool). Intensive Care Med 2009;35:890–8.
79. Sahuquillo J, Mena MP, Vilalta A, et al. Moderate hypothemia in the management of severe traumatic brain injury: a good idea proved ineffective? Curr Pharm Des 2004;10:2193–204.

Neurocritical Care

Status Epilepticus Review

Fawaz Al-Mufti, MD, Jan Claassen, MD, PhD, FNCS*

KEYWORDS

- Status epilepticus • Convulsions • Nonconvulsive • Treatment
- Continuous electroencephalogram monitoring • Intensive care unit
- Refractory status epilepticus

KEY POINTS

- Control seizures as soon as possible and do not undertreat.
- Determine the underlying cause of seizures rapidly and address this if possible.
- Once convulsions have ceased consider NCSz.

INTRODUCTION

Status epilepticus (SE) is a life-threatening medical and neurologic emergency that requires prompt diagnosis and treatment. SE may be classified into convulsive and nonconvulsive, based on the presence of rhythmic jerking of the extremities. Refractory status epilepticus (RSE) is defined as ongoing seizures failing to respond to first- and second-line anticonvulsant drug therapies. Among RSE patients, 10% to 15% fail to respond to third-line therapy, and are considered to have super-refractory SE (SRSE). Patients with SRSE are not well studied, and in the absence of randomized clinical trials, treatment is controversial.

SE is defined as convulsions lasting for 5 or more minutes or recurrent episodes of convulsions in a 5-minute interval without return to preconvulsive neurologic baseline. A typical secondarily generalized tonic–clonic seizure generally stops by 3 minutes and almost always by 5 minutes.[1]

Patients with nonconvulsive SE (NCSE) do not exhibit overt signs of convulsions but have seizure activity documented on electroencephalogram (EEG).

Treatment efficacy, morbidity, and mortality are directly related to delays in starting therapy.

Columbia University College of Physicians & Surgeons, 177 Fort Washington Avenue, Milstein 8 Center Room 300, New York, NY 10032, USA
* Corresponding author.
E-mail address: jc1439@columbia.edu

Crit Care Clin 30 (2014) 751–764
http://dx.doi.org/10.1016/j.ccc.2014.06.006
0749-0704/14/$ – see front matter © 2014 Elsevier Inc. All rights reserved.

Level of consciousness should start to improve within 20 minutes of cessation of the convulsions. If mental status remains abnormal for 30 to 60 minutes after the convulsions cease, NCSE must be considered, and urgent EEG is advised.

EPIDEMIOLOGY

SE accounts for 20% of emergency department visits for neurologic problems and 1% of all emergency department visits,[2–4] with a 9% to 27% 30-day mortality rate.[5]

Following the apparent resolution of clinical seizures, nonconvulsive electrographic seizures (NCSz) persist in 20% to 48% of patients, and 14% of patients are in NCSE without any clinical signs of seizure activity.

In neurologic intensive care units (ICUs), up to one-third of patients will have NCSz, and most of these patients will be in NCSE.

In medical ICU settings, the incidence of NCSE is estimated to be near 10%,[6] and it is particularly prevalent in patients with sepsis.[7]

RSE occurs in 30% to 43% of patients with SE.[8]

DIAGNOSIS AND CLINICAL PRESENTATION

Patients with generalized tonic–clonic status epilepticus (GCSE) present with continuous or repeated generalized tonic–clonic movements or rhythmic jerking of the extremities. Patients also exhibit alteration in their mental status ranging from decreased attentiveness and impaired responsiveness to a deep comatose state between convulsions. After convulsions have ceased, focal findings such as a focal motor impairment, also known as Todd paralysis, may persist.

NCSE has been described as electroclinical dissociation whereby patients may have ictal discharges on EEG, with or without subtle convulsive movements that may include twitching of the arms, legs, trunk, or facial muscles, tonic eye deviation, and nystagmoid eye jerking.

Psychogenic nonepileptic SE needs to be included in the differential diagnosis in patients who demonstrate poorly coordinated limb thrashing, back arching, pelvic thrusting, forced eye closure, head rolling, and preserved consciousness or purposeful movements. It is crucial to note that when in doubt, patients should be expeditiously treated as if they have SE.

DIFFERENTIAL DIAGNOSIS

Conditions to consider for the differential diagnosis include movement disorders (myoclonus, asterixis, tremor, chorea, tics, dystonia); herniation (decerebrate or decorticate posturing); Limb-shaking transient ischemic attacks, most commonly associated with perfusion failure due to severe carotid stenosis; psychiatric disorders (eg, psychogenic nonepileptic seizures, conversion disorder, acute psychosis, or catatonia); postanoxic myoclonus; or any condition that may lead to decreased level of consciousness (eg, toxic metabolic encephalopathies, including hypoglycemia and delirium, anoxia, and central nervous system [CNS] infections), transient global amnesia, sleep disorders (eg, parasomnias), and syncope.

DIAGNOSTIC WORK-UP

The diagnostic work-up should be conducted in parallel with treatment. Following are guidelines published by the Neurocritical Care Society for the evaluation and management of SE all patients should receive:[9]

- Fingerstick glucose
- Vital sign monitoring
- Head computed tomography (CT) scan (appropriate for most cases)
- Laboratory tests: blood glucose, complete blood count, basic metabolic panel, calcium (total and ionized), magnesium, antiepileptic drug (AED) levels.
- Continuous electroencephalogram (EEG) monitoring must be considered in all patients who do not return to clinical baseline (**Fig. 1**).

Comatose patients should undergo a minimum of 48 hours of 21-electrode EEG monitoring while those who are not comatose may only require 24 hours.

Patients whose EEGs demonstrate periodic epileptiform discharges may also require prolonged monitoring, since these patients may develop electrographic seizures.

The work-up should be tailored to the clinical scenario and in certain circumstances may require

- Brain magnetic resonance imaging (MRI)
- Lumbar puncture (LP): the presence of fever at presentation should raise the suspicion for CNS infection, and empiric treatment with bacterial and viral coverage should be started until the results from the LP and imaging ancillary testing are available
- Comprehensive toxicology panel including toxins that frequently cause seizures (ie, isoniazid, tricyclic antidepressants, theophylline, cocaine, sympathomimetics, alcohol, organophosphates, and cyclosporine)

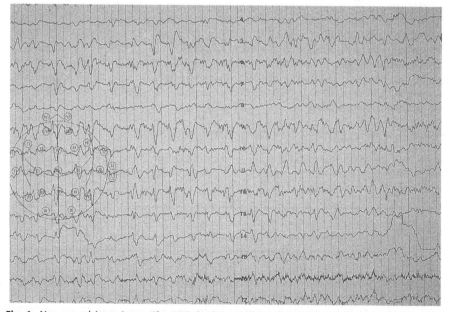

Fig. 1. Nonconvulsive seizure. The EEG depicts an electrographic seizure in a patient who is unresponsive but has no other clinical phenomena to suggest a seizure. At times, comatose patients may exhibit subtle eyelid or facial twitching or other subtle clinical signs. (*Courtesy of* C. Chang, MD, Honolulu, Hawaii.)

- Other laboratory tests: liver function tests, serial troponins, type and screen, coagulation studies, arterial blood gas, AED levels, toxicology screen (urine and blood), and inborn errors of metabolism
- Benzodiazepine trial: sequential small doses of rapidly acting, short-duration benzodiazepines (eg, midazolam 1 mg) are administered. Although rarely helpful, the resolution of the potentially ictal EEG pattern and either an improvement in the clinical state or the appearance of previously absent normal EEG patterns would be considered a positive response. If EEG improves, but the patient does not (eg, because of marked sedation), the result is equivocal

ACUTE MANAGEMENT OF SE

The most decisive element of therapy determining successful termination of seizures is the time elapsed before initiating benzodiazepines.

When treatment with intravenous agents is initiated within 30 minutes of seizure onset, the initial AED is successful in terminating SE patients' seizures in 80% of cases, whereas only 40% of patients respond to therapy started beyond the 2-hour window.[10] Furthermore, mortality doubles with a 24 hour delay in treatment of NCSE.[10]

PREHOSPITAL TREATMENT

Upon diagnosis, SE patients should receive benzodiazepine treatment either as intravenous administration of lorazepam (4 mg given over 2 minutes intravenously) or diazepam (5 mg intravenously), although alternate routes of administration are also possible, including 20 mg of diazepam per rectum, and intranasal, buccal, or intramuscular administration of 10 mg of midazolam.

First responders should be prepared to treat respiratory depression in patients with SE. Other important considerations for the prehospital management of SE include airway support, assuring stable circulation, obtaining intravenous access, and excluding hypoglycemia as a potential cause of SE.

Importantly, it was demonstrated that respiratory compromise was more commonly seen in patients who received placebo than those who were given benzodiazepines, suggesting that administering AEDs as soon as possible is not only more efficacious but also safer than waiting.[5]

INITIAL IN-HOSPITAL/EMERGENCY DEPARTMENT TREATMENT

Immediate attention should be directed at supporting the airway, breathing and circulation, obtaining intravenous access, and administering the first-line antiepileptic medication.

> Ongoing convulsions may be masked when using paralytics for intubation; therefore patients may continue to seize without any clinical manifestations.

SE caused by underlying metabolic abnormalities such as hypoglycemia is difficult to control with antiepileptic mediations and should be addressed specifically.

SE resulting from hypoglycemia should be treated promptly with 50 mL of D50W intravenously together with thiamine (100 mg intravenously).

Benzodiazepines should be given intravenously. If intravenous access cannot be established, benzodiazepine administration should not be delayed, and alternate routes of administration should be explored (eg, per rectum, buccal, intramuscular routes).

Although the initial benzodiazepine may stop the seizures, it is not a long-term therapy therefore all patients with GCSE should be given a first and second line AED simultaneously otherwise there is a high chance of SE recurrence.

SECONDARY IN-HOSPITAL TREATMENT

Phenytoin or fosphenytoin loading should be weight-based; hence fosphenytoin must be given at a dose of 20 mg/kg at 150 mg/min intravenously. If seizures persist, an additional 10 mg/kg at 150 mg/min may be given intravenously.

Hypotension may be seen with loading phenytoin or fosphenytoin in 28% to 50% of patients; therefore, loading should be performed with blood pressure and electrocardiogram monitoring. Do not adjust loading doses for renal or hepatic insufficiency.

Phenytoin loading should be weight based and the common practice of loading 1 g for everyone is incorrect and should be discontinued.

Phenytoin loading dose should not be adjusted for renal or hepatic insufficiency.

Valproic acid is an efficacious second-line treatment, associated with seizure abortion in 66% of patients.[11] Valproic acid is administered as 20 to 40 mg/kg over 10 minutes intravenously, with an additional 20 mg/kg subsequently over 5 minutes if the patient is still seizing (**Fig. 2**).

Valproic acid serum levels may be obtained immediately following the loading dose infusion, whereas phenytoin levels should be drawn 2 hours after the infusion of fosphenytoin or phenytoin.

Levetiracetam, loaded 2.5 g intravenously over 5 minutes or 1 to 4 g over 15 minutes, is often used off-label as a second-line agent but data are limited so far.[12]

Phenobarbital is US Food and Drug Administration (FDA) labeled for the treatment of SE, but it is less commonly chosen in adults unless other agents are contraindicated or unavailable. Phenobarbital 20 mg/kg is loaded intravenously at a rate of up to 50 to 100 mg/min, with an additional 5 to 10 mg/kg given if needed.

Lacosamide given intravenously as a bolus dose of 200 to 400 mg over 3 to 5 minutes may have some efficacy as an adjunctive agent in the treatment of status epilepticus;[13–15] however, this is still controversial.[16]

In patients in whom convulsions persist after the initial benzodiazepines, experts increasingly recommend skipping second-line antiepileptic medications and starting continuous antiepileptic medications such as midazolam or propofol.

Patients who do not return to their preconvulsive neurologic baseline within 20 minutes should be connected to EEG monitoring to diagnose subclinical electrographic seizures.

Although it is unclear how aggressive nonconvulsive electrographic seizures and nonconvulsive SE should be treated, most experts agree that in the acute brain injury setting, electrographic seizures should be treated aggressively.

- Clinical diagnosis; ABCs, establish intravenous access, cardiac telemetry monitoring; draw laboratory tests
- Thiamine 100 mg and D50W 50 ml IV
- Lorazepam 0.05 mg/kg (approximately 4 mg) / 2 min IV

↓

- Fosphenytoin load 20 mg/kg IV at up to 150 mg/min

  or
- Valproate acid load: 40 mg/kg IV over 10 min)
- If possible connect to EEG unless patient wakes up or returns to pre-convulsive baseline

↓

- Continuous intravenous infusion of midazolam or propofol
- Alternatively IV Valproate acid load: 40 mg/kg IV over 10 min
- Continuous EEG needed

↓

- Continuous intravenous infusion of pentobarbital (dosing see Box 1)
- cEEG needed

Fig. 2. Simplified outline for management of SE. ABCs, airway-breathing-circulation.

ADVANCED MANAGEMENT OF RSE

SE not responding to the initial 2 or more anticonvulsants should be considered to be in RSE regardless of the elapsed time. An aggressive treatment approach is required.

It is important to make the determination of refractoriness early (30–60 min), because delayed attempts to control SE with antiepileptic agents are frequently ineffective.

RSE patients are generally comatose, have cardiopulmonary compromise, and have associated systemic complications; hence they are best managed in an ICU setting.

> All second-line antiepileptic medications should be continued while treatment with continuous intravenous AED infusions is initiated.

Most experts recommend treatment with a continuous intravenous AED such as midazolam or propofol (**Box 1**) as the initial step in treating RSE.

Valproic acid, if not given earlier, may be a reasonable alternative especially in patients who have an active "do not intubate" order.

MIDAZOLAM

Midazolam is administered as 0.2 mg/kg followed by 0.2 to 0.4 mg/kg boluses every 5 minutes until seizures stop, up to a maximum total loading dose of 2 mg/kg.[9]

Maintenance infusion should be initiated upon seizure control at a rate of 0.05 to 2.9 mg/kg/h. Among midazolam's advantages are its rapid onset, easy titration, greater water solubility, and circumvention of the metabolic acidosis associated with the propylene glycol vehicle of other benzodiazepines and barbiturates.[9,17,18]

Box 1
Treatment of RSE

Midazolam

- Load: 0.2 mg/kg intravenously over 2 to 5 minutes; repeat 0.2 to 0.4 mg/kg boluses every 5 minutes until seizures stop, up to a maximum loading dose of 2 mg/kg.
- Initial rate: 0.1 mg/kg/h; bolus and increase rate until seizure control
- Maintenance: 0.05 to 2.9 mg/kg/h

Propofol

- Load: 1 to 2 mg/kg intravenously over 3 to 5 minutes; repeat boluses every 3 to 5 minutes until seizures stop, up to maximum total loading dose of 10 mg/kg.
- Initial rate: 20 µg/kg/min; bolus and increase rate until seizure control
- Maintenance: 30 to 200 µg/kg/min titrated to EEG with 5 to 10 µg/kg/min every 5 min or 1 mg/kg bolus for breakthrough SE

Valproic acid

- 20 to 40 mg/kg intravenously over 10 minutes (may give additional 20 mg/kg over 5 minutes if seizures persist)

Pentobarbital

- Load: 5 to 15 mg/kg (5–10 mg/kg in patients with pre-existing hypotension) infused over 1 hour; may repeat 5 mg/kg boluses until seizures stop.
- Initial rate: 1 mg/kg/h
- Maintenance: 0.5 to 5 mg/kg/h, titrated to maintain seizure suppression pattern on EEG and a serum level of 30 to 45 µg/mL; for breakthrough SE, a 5 mg/kg bolus must be given, and the continuous infusion rate should be increased by 0.5 to 1 mg/kg/h every 12 hours

Ketamine

- The optimum dose in refractory SE is uncertain but has been extrapolated from the anesthesia literature (1–4.5 mg/kg with supplements of 0.5–2.5 mg/kg every 30–45 min or 10–50 µg/kg/min).
- Load: 1.5 mg/kg every 3 to 5 minutes until seizure stops, up to a maximum of 4.5 mg/kg
- Initial rate: 20 µg/kg/minutes (1.2 mg/kg/h; bolus and increase rate by 10–20 µg/kg/min until seizure control is established)
- Maintenance: 5 to 125 µg/kg/min (0.3–7.5 mg/kg/h)

Its major disadvantages include the short half-life requiring a continuous infusion and the development of tachyphylaxis with prolonged infusions.[19] Several reports have demonstrated its efficacy in RSE.[20,21]

Patients with refractory NCSE treated with continuous infusions of midazolam were found to have acute treatment failure and breakthrough seizures in 18% and 56% of patients, respectively[22]

A recent study compared adults with RSE treated with high-dose continuous intravenous midazolam with those treated with the previous lower-dose continuous intravenous midazolam. Compared with the low-dose group, high-dose continuous intravenous midazolam treatment of RSE was associated with a lower seizure rate after midazolam discontinuation (15% vs 64%), and it may be associated with lower mortality than traditional lower-dose protocols. Hypotension was more frequent with higher continuous intravenous midazolam doses, but this was not associated with worse outcome.[18]

PROPOFOL

The Neurocritical Care Society guidelines on SE recommend starting a propofol drip at 20 µg/kg/min, with a 1 to 2 mg/kg loading dose followed by continuous infusion dosing at 30 to 200 µg/kg/min titrated to EEG, with 5 to 10 µg/kg/min every 5 min or 1 mg/kg bolus for breakthrough SE.[9]

Propofol's onset of action is within 3 to 5 minutes, and activity persists only for 5 to 10 minutes after discontinuation. Significant concerns when using propofol include respiratory suppression, hypotension, infections with prolonged infusions, and propofol infusion syndrome (PRIS). PRIS is a rare but potentially lethal complication characterized clinically by dysrhythmia (eg, bradycardia or tachycardia), heart failure, hyperkalemia, hypertriglyceridemia, metabolic acidosis, and rhabdomyolysis or myoglobinuria with subsequent renal failure[23] and death.

Because propofol is delivered in a lipid vehicle, some advocate adjustment of dietary calories to avoid overfeeding. Rapid discontinuation should be avoided, as it may precipitate withdrawal seizures.[24]

Advantages of propofol include less tachyphylaxis than midazolam and less hypotension than pentobarbital.[25] Both midazolam and propofol are more expensive than high-dose barbiturates. There do not seem to be significant cost differences between the 2 drugs.

BARBITURATES

Continuous intravenous infusions of pentobarbital, a mainstay of RSE treatment for the past 50 years, has been used less frequently as third-line therapy in favor of midazolam or propofol.

Pentobarbital is administered with a loading dose of 5 to 15 mg/kg (5–10 mg/kg in patients with pre-existing hypotension) infused over 1 hour, followed by an initial maintenance continuous infusion at a rate of 0.5 to 5 mg/kg/h, titrated to maintain seizure suppression pattern on EEG that corresponds typically with a serum level of 30 to 45 µg/mL. For breakthrough SE, a 5 mg/kg bolus must be given, and the continuous infusion rate should be increased by 0.5 to 1 mg/kg/h every 12 hours.[9,26]

Hypotension is frequently seen as an adverse effect of pentobarbital, and vasopressors should be readily available. Other adverse effects include gastric stasis, myocardial suppression, thrombocytopenia, and metabolic acidosis.

The main limitations of pentobarbital's use are related to the adverse effect profile that includes hypotension requiring pressors,[27] prolonged mechanical ventilation,[28] very long half-life (15–50 hours), blood dyscrasias, and allergic reactions ranging from angioedema to Stevens-Johnson syndrome. It must be used with caution in patients with hepatic or renal impairment. Furthermore, high-dose barbiturates are potentially immunosuppressive, and extra care is needed to prevent and treat nosocomial infections.[29]

As mentioned previously, when comparing treatment of RSE with continuous infusions of propofol, midazolam, or pentobarbital, mortality at discharge was not different.[17] By contrast, pentobarbital had a lower frequency of acute treatment failure and breakthrough seizures.

A recent paper on super refractory SE showed that pentobarbital drips controlled seizures in 90% of patients. Although seizures recurred in 48% of patients while weaning, 80% of those patients were eventually weaned successfully, many with the addition of phenobarbital given enterally. The retrospective analysis also found fewer adverse effects (ventilator-associated pneumonia, hypotension, urinary tract infections) compared with previously published data.[30]

KETAMINE

The optimum dose of ketamine in RSE is uncertain but has been extrapolated from the anesthesia literature. An initial 1.5 mg/kg loading dose is given every 3 to 5 minutes until seizure stop (maximum dose of 4.5 mg/kg). The initial infusion rate is 20 μg/kg/min (1.2 mg/kg/h), but if seizure control is not established, a bolus should be given, and rate should be increased by 10–20 μg/kg/min. Patients are kept on maintenance rate of 5 to 125 μg/kg/min (0.3–7.5 mg/kg/h).

As excitatory N-methyl-D-aspartate (NMDA) receptors are upregulated with prolonged SE, NMDA receptor (NMDAR) antagonists such as ketamine are attractive as a potential treatment for RSE.[31]

A recently published systematic literature review regarding the use of NMDAR antagonists for RSE described 110 adult patients, and showed electroencephalographic seizure control in 56.5% of patients, with a 63.5% response in the 52 pediatric patients described.[32]

Moreover, ketamine appears to have a synergistic effect when combined with benzodiazepines.[33,34]

Adverse events have been rare, and overall ketamine appears to be a relatively effective and safe drug for the treatment of RSE. However, unlike most of the other agents used for RSE, it causes elevation of the blood pressure.

Caution is warranted in patients with elevated intracranial pressure, traumatic brain injury (TBI), ocular injuries, hypertension, chronic congestive heart failure (CHF), myocardial infarction (MI), tachyarrhythmias, and history of alcohol abuse.[35] Further prospective study of early ketamine administration is warranted.

Less well-studied approaches to control RSE include medications that target refractoriness of SE to therapies that may be neuroprotective (ie, therapeutic hypothermia). All of these have been poorly studied and at this point should be considered investigational (**Box 2**).

The exact mechanisms underlying the development of refractoriness are incompletely understood. Evidence has accumulated that impairment of gamma-aminobutyric acid (GABA)–mediated inhibition related to internalization of GABA receptors[17,36–39] and upregulation of excitatory AMPA (alpha-amino-3-hydroxy-5-methyl-4-isoxazolepropionate) and NMDA (N-methyl-D-aspartate) receptors[38] may play a role in the development of increasing refractoriness to treatment.

TREATMENT ENDPOINTS

Controversy exists regarding the electrographic target of continuous drips. Some advocate for seizure suppression; others prefer burst suppression or even complete background suppression.

Once control of SE is achieved with at least 1 of the previously mentioned medications, many experts continue continuous intravenous AED therapy for 24 to 48 hours

---

Box 2
Alternative therapies RSE

Pharmacologic

- Ketamine
- Corticosteroids
- Inhaled anesthetics
- Immunomodulation (intravenous immunoglobulin or plasmaphoresis)

Nonpharmacological

- Vagus nerve stimulation
- Ketogenic diet
- Hypothermia
- Electroconvulsive therapy
- Transcranial magnetic stimulation
- Surgical management

Case reports and small case series

- Lidocaine
- Verapamil
- Paraldehyde
- Acetazolamide
- Deep brain stimulation

---

of complete seizure control before gradually withdrawing the antiepileptic/anesthetic drug infusions, but this is based mostly on expert consensus. Weaning should be done while the patient is under EEG monitoring.

Simultaneously, maintenance doses of traditional anticonvulsants should be continued to facilitate withdrawal of anesthetic drug infusions.

Withdrawal seizures may be seen in approximately half of the patients and should be treated promptly. Some advocate restarting the continuous intravenous AED at the rate that the patient was on prior to the taper; others opt to add some of the second-line AEDs that were not used earlier and then repeat tapering after 24 hours without seizures. Alternatively patients may be switched to a different continuous AED.

COMPLICATIONS

SE is a multisystem disease affecting most organs of the body requiring ICU level of care. Most organs can be secondarily affected by ongoing seizure activity or as a consequence of treatment.

Neurology

Prolonged or repetitive seizures reach a point when they are unlikely to end spontaneously, and hence in addition to causing brain injury, they are associated with higher mortality and worse clinical outcomes.[22,40–42]

Continuous seizures lasting more than 20 to 30 minutes have been associated with irreversible cerebral injury[43] and pharmacoresistance.[39,44]

The presence of cortical laminar necrosis, representing neuronal death, apparent on magnetic resonance imaging (MRI), has been correlated clinically with increasing neurologic morbidity with increasing seizure duration, even after the effects of etiology are eliminated.[42,45]

Cardiac

Cardiac arrhythmias are frequently seen in ongoing SE. Stress cardiomyopathy with contraction band necrosis, presumably secondary to massive catecholamine release, has been associated with death during SE.

Pulmonary

Many patients with SE and most with RSE may be unable to protect their airways and hence warrant intubation. Hypoxia, pulmonary edema, and aspiration are frequently seen.

Infectious Disease

Infections may precipitate SE (meningitis, encephalitis) and may develop secondary to SE as in pneumonias. Any fever in a patient with SE should be worked up expeditiously. Blood, urine, and cerebrospinal fluid cultures, as well as a chest radiograph, may be necessary. It should be noted that a mild elevation in white blood cell count may be seen in the serum and cerebrospinal fluid (CSF) as a consequence of ongoing seizure activity.

Electrolytes

Metabolic derangements (glucose, sodium, phosphate, calcium, pH) can be the underlying cause or the effect of SE. These should be corrected aggressively as outlined previously, since seizures may be very difficult to control with persistent metabolic abnormalities.

Renal

Renal failure due to rhabdomyolysis and myoglobinuria may be seen after prolonged convulsive SE and should be treated with adequate hydration.

PROGNOSIS

Overall, despite medical interventions, in-hospital mortality associated with SE ranges between 9.4% and 21%,[5,46,47] and the 30-day mortality rate is between19% and 27%.[11,48–51]

Patients with prolonged SE beyond 1 hour, myoclonic SE, and symptomatic SE have higher mortality.[52]

RSE carries a poor outcome, with mortality rates between 23% and 61%,[17,22,47,53–55] and it appears to be independent of the chosen therapeutic strategy. In a large retrospective case series on SRSE, patients were found to have a mortality rate of 42%, which is higher than previously described for SE.

In-hospital mortality of patients with NCSE is between 18% and 52% and goes up to 65% at 1-month follow-up.

Although etiology is the most important predictor of outcome, older age, medical comorbidity, and high initial APACHE (Acute Physiology and Chronic Health Evaluation) scores are also independent risk factors for mortality.[38,56–58]

SE secondary to noncompliance or abrupt discontinuation of AEDs, head trauma, and alcohol withdrawal has good outcome in 90% of patients, whereas older age, impairment of consciousness, duration of SE, the presence of medical complications and etiologies such as stroke, acute metabolic dysfunction, and anoxia have a poorer outcome.[46,59,60]

SE will recur in approximately one-third of patients, according to 1 population-based study that followed patients for 10 years.[61]

REFERENCES

1. Theodore WH, Porter RJ, Albert P, et al. The secondarily generalized tonic-clonic seizure: a videotape analysis. Neurology 1994;44(8):1403–7.
2. Claassen J, Silbergleit R, Weingart SD, et al. Emergency neurological life support: status epilepticus. Neurocrit Care 2012;17(Suppl 1):S73–8.
3. Pallin DJ, Goldstein JN, Moussally JS, et al. Seizure visits in US emergency departments: epidemiology and potential disparities in care. Int J Emerg Med 2008;1(2):97–105.
4. Pitts S, Niska RW, Xu J, et al. National Hospital Ambulatory Medical Care Survey: 2006 emergency department summary. Natl Health Stat Report 2008;6(7):1–38.
5. Alldredge BK, Gelb AM, Isaacs SM, et al. A comparison of lorazepam, diazepam, and placebo for the treatment of out-of-hospital status epilepticus. N Engl J Med 2001;345(9):631–7.
6. Young GB, Jordan KG, Doig GS. An assessment of nonconvulsive seizures in the intensive care unit using continuous EEG monitoring: an investigation of variables associated with mortality. Neurology 1996;47(1):83–9.
7. Oddo M, Carrera E, Claassen J, et al. Continuous electroencephalography in the medical intensive care unit. Crit Care Med 2009;37(6):2051–6.
8. Mayer SA, Claassen J, Lokin J, et al. Refractory status epilepticus: frequency, risk factors, and impact on outcome. Arch Neurol 2002;59(2):205–10.
9. Brophy GM, Bell R, Claassen J, et al. Guidelines for the evaluation and management of status epilepticus. Neurocrit Care 2012;17(1):3–23.
10. Lowenstein DH. Status epilepticus: an overview of the clinical problem. Epilepsia 1999;40(Suppl 1):S3–8 [discussion: S21–2].
11. Misra UK, Kalita J, Patel R. Sodium valproate vs phenytoin in status epilepticus: a pilot study. Neurology 2006;67(2):340–2.
12. Moddel G, Bunten S, Dobis C, et al. Intravenous levetiracetam: a new treatment alternative for refractory status epilepticus. J Neurol Neurosurg Psychiatry 2009; 80(6):689–92.
13. Albers JM, Möddel G, Dittrich R, et al. Intravenous lacosamide—an effective add-on treatment of refractory status epilepticus. Seizure 2011;20:428–30.
14. Kellinghaus C, Berning S, Immisch I, et al. Intravenous lacosamide for treatment of status epilepticus. Acta Neurol Scand 2011;123(2):137–41.
15. Höfler J, Trinka E. Lacosamide as a new treatment option in status epilepticus. Epilepsia 2013;54(3):393–404.
16. Goodwin H, Hinson HE, Shermock KM, et al. The use of lacosamide in refractory status epilepticus. Neurocrit Care 2011;14:348–53.
17. Claassen J, Hirsch LJ, Emerson RG, et al. Treatment of refractory status epilepticus with pentobarbital, propofol, or midazolam: a systematic review. Epilepsia 2002;43(2):146–53.
18. Fernandez A, Lantigua H, Lesch C, et al. High-dose midazolam infusion for refractory status epilepticus. Neurology 2014;82(4):359–65.
19. Shafer A. Complications of sedation with midazolam in the intensive care unit and a comparison with other sedative regimens. Crit Care Med 1998;26(5):947–56.

20. Igartua J, Silver P, Maytal J, et al. Midazolam coma for refractory status epilepticus in children. Crit Care Med 1999;27(9):1982–5.
21. Koul RL, Raj Aithala G, Chacko A, et al. Continuous midazolam infusion as treatment of status epilepticus. Arch Dis Child 1997;76(5):445–8.
22. Claassen J, Hirsch LJ, Emerson RG, et al. Continuous EEG monitoring and midazolam infusion for refractory nonconvulsive status epilepticus. Neurology 2001; 57(6):1036–42.
23. Kam PC, Cardone D. Propofol infusion syndrome. Anaesthesia 2007;62(7):690–701.
24. Finley GA, MacManus B, Sampson SE, et al. Delayed seizures following sedation with propofol. Can J Anaesth 1993;40(9):863–5.
25. Huff JS, Bleck TP. Propofol and midazolam in status epilepticus. Acad Emerg Med 1996;3(2):179.
26. Bleck T. Critical care medicine: principles of diagnosis and management. Chicago: Mosby-Year Book; 1995.
27. Yaffe K, Lowenstein DH. Prognostic factors of pentobarbital therapy for refractory generalized status epilepticus. Neurology 1993;43(5):895–900.
28. Rossetti AO, Milligan TA, Vulliemoz S, et al. A randomized trial for the treatment of refractory status epilepticus. Neurocrit Care 2011;14(1):4–10.
29. Devlin E, Clarke RS, Mirakhur RK, et al. Effect of four I.V. induction agents on T-lymphocyte proliferations to PHA in vitro. Br J Anaesth 1994;73(3):315–7.
30. Pugin D, Foreman B, De Marchis GM, et al. Is pentobarbital safe and efficacious in the treatment of super-refractory status epilepticus: a cohort study. Crit Care 2014;18:R103.
31. Kramer AH. Early ketamine to treat refractory status epilepticus. Neurocrit Care 2012;16(2):299–305.
32. Zeiler F, Teitelbaum J, Gillman LM. NMDA antagonists for refractory seizures. Neurocrit Care 2014;20:502–13.
33. Martin B, Kapur J. A combination of ketamine and diazepam synergistically controls refractory status epilepticus induced by cholinergic stimulation. Epilepsia 2008;49(2):248–55.
34. Hsieh C, Sung PS, Tsai JJ, et al. Terminating prolonged refractory status epilepticus using ketamine. Clin Neuropharmacol 2010;33(3):165–7.
35. Mewasingh L, Sékhara T, Aeby A, et al. Oral ketamine in paediatric nonconvulsive status epilepticus. Seizure 2003;12(7):483–9.
36. Naylor DE, Liu H, Wasterlain CG. Trafficking of GABAA receptors, loss of inhibition, and a mechanism for pharmacoresistance in status epilepticus. J Neurosci 2005;25:7724–33.
37. Meierkord H, Boon P, Engelsen B, et al. EFNS guideline on the management of status epilepticus. Eur J Neurol 2006;13(5):445–50.
38. Prasad A, Worrall BB, Bertram EH, et al. Propofol and midazolam in the treatment of refractory status epilepticus. Epilepsia 2001;42(3):380–6.
39. Chen JW, Wasterlain CG. Status epilepticus: pathophysiology and management in adults. Lancet Neurol 2006;5(3):246–56.
40. Legriel S, Bruneel F, Dalle L, et al. Recurrent takotsubo cardiomyopathy triggered by convulsive status epilepticus. Neurocrit Care 2008;9(1):118–21.
41. Legriel S, Azoulay E, Resche-Rigon M, et al. Functional outcome after convulsive status epilepticus. Crit Care Med 2010;38(12):2295–303.
42. Scholtes FB, Renier WO, Meinardi H. Generalized convulsive status epilepticus: causes, therapy, and outcome in 346 patients. Epilepsia 1994;35(5):1104–12.
43. Bleck T. Convulsive disorders: status epilepticus. Clin Neuropharmacol 1991;14: 191–8.

44. Mazarati AM, Baldwin RA, Sankar R, et al. Time-dependent decrease in the effectiveness of antiepileptic drugs during the course of self-sustaining status epilepticus. Brain Res 1998;814(1–2):179–85.
45. Payne T, Bleck TP. Status epilepticus. Crit Care Clin 1997;13(1):17–38.
46. Claassen J, Lokin JK, Fitzsimmons BF, et al. Predictors of functional disability and mortality after status epilepticus. Neurology 2002;58(1):139–42.
47. Novy J, Logroscino G, Rossetti AO. Refractory status epilepticus: a prospective observational study. Epilepsia 2010;51(2):251–6.
48. Logroscino G, Hesdorffer DC, Cascino G, et al. Short-term mortality after a first episode of status epilepticus. Epilepsia 1997;38(12):1344–9.
49. DeLorenzo R, Pellock JM, Towne AR, et al. Epidemiology of status epilepticus. J Clin Neurophysiol 1995;12(4):316–25.
50. Shorvon S. Status epilepticus: its clinical features and treatment in children and adults. Cambridge (England): Cambridge University Press; 1994.
51. Treiman DM, Meyers PD, Walton NY, et al. A comparison of four treatments for generalized convulsive status epilepticus. Veterans Affairs Status Epilepticus Cooperative Study Group. N Engl J Med 1998;339(12):792–8.
52. Logroscino G, Hesdorffer DC, Cascino GD, et al. Long-term mortality after a first episode of status epilepticus. Neurology 2002;58(4):537–41.
53. Krishnamurthy KB, Drislane FW. Depth of EEG suppression and outcome in barbiturate anesthetic treatment for refractory status epilepticus. Epilepsia 1999;40(6):759–62.
54. Stecker MM, Kramer TH, Raps EC, et al. Treatment of refractory status epilepticus with propofol: clinical and pharmacokinetic findings. Epilepsia 1998;39(1):18–26.
55. Rossetti AO, Reichhart MD, Schaller MD, et al. Propofol treatment of refractory status epilepticus: a study of 31 episodes. Epilepsia 2004;45(7):757–63.
56. Koubeissi M, Alshekhlee A. In-hospital mortality of generalized convulsive status epilepticus: a large US sample. Neurology 2007;69(9):886–93.
57. Rossetti AO, Hurwitz S, Logroscino G, et al. Prognosis of status epilepticus: role of aetiology, age, and consciousness impairment at presentation. J Neurol Neurosurg Psychiatry 2006;77(5):611–5.
58. Alvarez V, Januel JM, Burnand B, et al. Second-line status epilepticus treatment: comparison of phenytoin, valproate, and levetiracetam. Epilepsia 2011;52(7):1292–6.
59. Lowenstein DH, Alldredge BK. Status epilepticus at an urban public hospital in the 1980s. Neurology 1993;43(3 Pt 1):483–8.
60. Logroscino G, Hesdorffer DC, Cascino G, et al. Time trends in incidence, mortality, and case-fatality after first episode of status epilepticus. Epilepsia 2001;42(8):1031–5.
61. Hesdorffer D, Logroscino G, Cascino GD, et al. Recurrence of afebrile status epilepticus in a population-based study in Rochester, Minnesota. Neurology 2007;69(1):73–8.

Brain Resuscitation and Prognosis After Cardiac Arrest

Matthew A. Koenig, MD, FNCS

KEYWORDS

- Cardiac arrest • Hypoxic-ischemic encephalopathy • Induced hypothermia
- Prognostication • Coma

KEY POINTS

- Hyperoxia after cardiac arrest may worsen brain injury because of increased generation of reactive oxygen species.
- Targeted temperature management may improve outcomes after cardiac arrest but the latest clinical trial suggests that a target temperature of 36°C and fever avoidance are adequate.
- Most cardiac arrest patients do not require routine continuous EEG monitoring and ICP monitoring.
- Prognostic testing should be delayed until after rewarming and is most accurate with a combination of clinical and electrophysiologic tests.
- After induced hypothermia, recovery of awakening and motor responses may be delayed in patients with favorable outcomes.

INTRODUCTION

Most patients who are admitted to an intensive care unit (ICU) after successful resuscitation from cardiac arrest are comatose and have uncertain prognosis. Aggressive management often requires invasive procedures, complex hemodynamic support, and several days of brain-directed treatment before the prognosis becomes clear. Outcomes are often disappointing and providers and families are left to struggle with difficult decisions regarding goals of care, acceptable outcomes, and end-of-life decisions. Treatment of cardiac arrest survivors can be unrewarding, which may

---

Disclosure Statement: Dr M. Koenig received grant support for research in brain injury related to cardiac arrest as a sub-investigator on NIH COBRE 1P30GM103341-01 (PI: Shohet), principal investigator of Hawaii Community Foundation grant # 11ADVC-49231, and through the Queen Emma Research Fund. No other relevant disclosures.
The Queen's Medical Center, Neuroscience Institute, 1301 Punchbowl Street, QET5, Honolulu, HI 96813, USA
E-mail address: mkoenig@queens.org

Crit Care Clin 30 (2014) 765–783
http://dx.doi.org/10.1016/j.ccc.2014.06.007
0749-0704/14/$ – see front matter © 2014 Elsevier Inc. All rights reserved.

criticalcare.theclinics.com

result in clinical pessimism and self-fulfilling prophesies. Over the last decade, the apparent success of induced hypothermia to improve neurologic outcomes after cardiac arrest has been one major beacon of hope. The latest clinical trial data, however, failed to show a benefit for induced hypothermia over maintenance of normothermia in cardiac arrest survivors. This article reviews the contemporary management of cardiac arrest with a particular focus on brain-directed therapies and the latest information on prognostication and neuromonitoring.

EPIDEMIOLOGY AND IMPACT

In the United States, the annual incidence of nontraumatic, out-of-hospital cardiac arrest is around 350,000 or 80 per 100,000 adults.[1] Although the incidence of out-of-hospital cardiac arrest with a shockable initial rhythm seems to be decreasing, the incidence of cardiac arrest with any initial rhythm has been static.[1] Despite the increasing availability of automated external defibrillators, cardiopulmonary resuscitation (CPR) training among the lay public, and advances in postresuscitation care, the survival and functional outcomes after cardiac arrest remain poor. Only 9.5% of patients with out-of-hospital cardiac arrest survive to hospital discharge.[1] Hypoxic-ischemic brain injury and withdrawal of life-sustaining treatment are a major cause of mortality. Functional outcomes among cardiac arrest survivors are also typically poor with brain injury representing a major mechanism of long-term disability.[2] Cognitive dysfunction and memory impairment contribute to the inability to return to full-time employment for most cardiac arrest survivors.[2] Functional independence rates and health-related quality of life have also been reported as poor in the most outcome studies.[2]

PATHOPHYSIOLOGY OF BRAIN INJURY AFTER CARDIAC ARREST

Unlike stroke, cardiac arrest produces brain injury through transient global loss of cerebral perfusion, followed by a period of global hypoperfusion during CPR. After return of spontaneous circulation (ROSC), cerebral perfusion is restored. During the period of total circulatory arrest, ATP production ceases within seconds, which leads to rapid dysfunction of ATP-dependent sodium-potassium pumps on the neuronal membrane.[3] This process leads to disruption of the blood-brain barrier, intracellular acidosis, and neuronal edema.[3] Glutamate-mediated excitotoxicity and a rise in intracellular calcium also contribute to the early stages of apoptotic cell death.[3] In addition, stasis of blood within the cerebral vasculature results in formation of microthrombi, which impede reperfusion after ROSC.[3] Ischemic injury to the endothelium and early activation of neutrophils also contribute to ongoing damage to the cerebral microvasculature.[3] These factors contribute to reperfusion failure that increases with the duration of cardiac arrest, the "no-reflow" phenomenon.[3]

During CPR, there is partial restoration of cerebral perfusion and oxygenation. Increased perfusion also means increased delivery of reactive oxygen species, inflammatory mediators, cytokines, and neutrophils, which contribute to secondary neuronal injury.[3] After ROSC, there is loss of cerebral autoregulation resulting in regional and temporal disparities in cerebral perfusion with some brain regions experiencing ongoing hypoperfusion, whereas others are relatively hyperperfused. Hypoperfusion may result in ongoing ischemic neuronal death, whereas hyperperfusion contributes to edema and secondary neuronal injury.[3] These regional disparities in post-ROSC perfusion may partially account for the selective vulnerability of specific brain regions to global hypoxic-ischemic events.

Ischemic neuronal injury is not observed for several hours after ROSC and the demonstration of typical histologic markers of ischemia (**Fig. 1**) is strongly associated with the interval between ROSC and autopsy.[4] Patients who survive for several days after ROSC are more likely to demonstrate extensive ischemic neuronal injury on autopsy.[4] Selective vulnerability to global hypoxia-ischemia has been observed in the projection neurons residing in the deep layers of the cerebral cortex, cerebellar Purkinje cells, and the CA-1 sector of the hippocampus.[5] Subcortical regions, white matter, and nonneuronal support cells are relatively resistant to short periods of global cerebral hypoxia-ischemia.[5] Progressive injury to thalamic and cortical neurons contributes to disorders of consciousness that are frequently observed among survivors of cardiac arrest.[6] Selective vulnerability of the hippocampus results in the memory dysfunction commonly found in cardiac arrest survivors with cognitive deficits.[6]

Ischemic stroke injures all tissues within a perfusion bed and is rapidly conspicuous on brain imaging. Conversely, selective neuronal injury from cardiac arrest results in relatively bland findings on early brain imaging with poor sensitivity for brain injury. Progressive cerebral atrophy is noted more chronically.[7] Loss of gray matter volume is particularly demonstrable in the anterior, medial, and posterior cingulate cortex; the precuneus; insular cortex; posterior hippocampus; and the dorsomedial thalamus.[7] Selective atrophy of these structures is associated with disorders of consciousness, cognitive dysfunction, and memory deficits observed in long-term survivors of cardiac arrest.[6]

PREHOSPITAL STABILIZATION AND EVALUATION OF CARDIAC ARREST

Postresuscitation care requires complex, multidisciplinary treatment. High-volume centers with experience in caring for cardiac arrest survivors, established protocols, and tertiary services provide optimal care.[8] The American Heart Association (AHA) has issued guidelines for postresuscitation care, including the immediate prehospital period.[8] These recommendations include securing the airway for patients with poor airway protective reflexes caused by depressed level of consciousness. Emergency medical services providers are also instructed to maintain the head of bed elevated

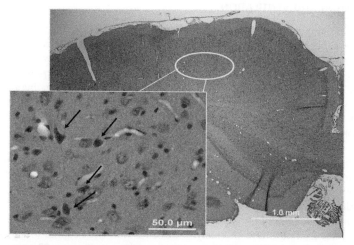

Fig. 1. Hematoxylin and eosin stain showing ischemic neuronal death with pyknotic, eosinophilic neurons (*arrows*) identified in the cerebral cortex of a rat 72 hours after resuscitation from cardiac arrest.

to reduce the impact of cerebral edema.[8] Ventilation and oxygenation strategies may also impact neuronal injury after cardiac arrest. Excessive ventilation may cause cerebral ischemia from cerebral vasoconstriction, and excessive oxygenation contributes to neuronal injury through generation of reactive oxygen species.[8] For these reasons, the AHA guidelines recommend titration of supplemental oxygen to maintain saturation only greater than or equal to 94% and minute ventilation to maintain $Paco_2$ of 40 to 45 mm Hg.[8] The optimal blood pressure target for cardiac arrest survivors is not known; however, guidelines were devised to balance the risk of exacerbating reperfusion injury and cerebral edema from hypertension against the risk of worsening cerebral ischemia from hypotension. Current AHA guidelines recommend maintaining a systolic blood pressure greater than or equal to 90 mm Hg and mean arterial pressure greater than or equal to 65 mm Hg.[8]

ANGIOGRAPHY AND CORONARY INTERVENTION

Patients with high clinical suspicion of acute coronary syndromes should undergo revascularization in tandem with other therapies, including targeted temperature management, if indicated.[8] Although clinical trials have not been undertaken to test the effectiveness of early coronary angiography and percutaneous coronary intervention (PCI) in cardiac arrest survivors, a growing number of observational studies have suggested a benefit.[9] In patients without an obvious noncardiac cause for cardiac arrest, the reported prevalence of significant coronary artery disease ranged from 59% to 71%.[9] A recent single-center observational study reported outcomes of initially comatose patients resuscitated from cardiac arrest who underwent immediate coronary angiography and PCI, if indicated.[10] Survival to discharge occurred in 32% of the overall cohort, but was higher in patients with documented acute coronary syndromes as the cause of cardiac arrest.[10] Among those who survived to hospital discharge, 82% remained alive after 5 years of follow-up.[10] Until clinical trial results are available, these observational data argue for consideration of PCI in cardiac arrest survivors (especially in the setting of suspected acute coronary syndromes) even among patients who are initially comatose.

OXYGENATION AND VENTILATION

There is mounting evidence for cautious management of oxygenation and ventilation in comatose cardiac arrest survivors. In a large, multicenter cohort study of 6326 patients admitted to ICUs at 120 US hospitals after resuscitation from cardiac arrest, a strong association was found between arterial blood gas findings within the first 24 hours of admission and in-hospital mortality.[11] In this study, hyperoxia was defined by Pao_2 greater than or equal to 300 mm Hg and hypoxia was defined as Pao_2 less than or equal to 60 mm Hg within the first 24 hours of ICU admission. In this cohort, 18% had hyperoxia and 19% had hypoxia. The in-hospital mortality was 63% in the hyperoxia group, 57% in the hypoxia group, and 45% in the normoxia group with an odds ratio for death of 1.8 for the hyperoxia group after for controlling for potential confounders.[11] Another recent multicenter cohort study did not find an association between hyperoxia within the first 24 hours after resuscitation from cardiac arrest and neurologic outcomes at 12 months.[12] A recent cohort study of children resuscitated from cardiac arrest found an association between $Paco_2$ within the first 24 hours and mortality.[13] Patients with hypocapnia ($Paco_2$ <30 mm Hg) had a mortality of 50%, and those with hypercapnia ($Paco_2$ >50 mm Hg) had a mortality of 59%. These patients had a significantly higher mortality than normocapnic patients (mortality of 33%).[13] Although the exact oxygenation and ventilation targets need to be identified, these studies highlight the importance of avoiding hyperoxia, hypercapnia, and hypocapnia during the acute period after resuscitation from cardiac arrest.

BLOOD PRESSURE MANAGEMENT

Arterial hypotension may worsen brain injury after cardiac arrest because of ongoing cerebral hypoperfusion. Using a database of 120 US ICUs, data were examined for 8736 patients admitted after resuscitation from cardiac arrest.[14] Hypotension was defined as one or more systolic blood pressure readings less than 90 mm Hg within 1 hour of arrival to the ICU. Hypotension was present in nearly half of included patients.[14] Not surprisingly, mortality was higher (65%) among patients with hypotension after ROSC compared with 37% mortality in normotensive patients.[14] Data are currently absent regarding the safe upper limits of blood pressure after cardiac arrest. However, because cerebral autoregulation is disrupted acutely, the relationship between arterial hypertension and intracranial pressure (ICP) and cerebral edema formation is expected to be linear. For this reason, severe hypertension and cerebral hyperperfusion would be expected to contribute to intracranial hypertension and cerebral edema. The current AHA guidelines recommend maintenance of systolic blood pressure greater than or equal to 90 mm Hg and mean arterial pressure greater than or equal to 65 mm Hg.[8] Until more precise data are available, maintenance of systolic blood pressure less than 160 mm Hg after ROSC also seems reasonable to limit cerebral hyperperfusion.

GLYCEMIC CONTROL

Appropriate target glycemic control after cardiac arrest is another source of uncertainty. Because glucose is the primary source of energy for neuronal metabolism and the brain has no mechanism for glucose storage, hypoglycemia could contribute to metabolic failure and worsened neuronal injury after cardiac arrest. However, hyperglycemia has been consistently associated with poor outcomes after ischemic stroke in humans and animal data have demonstrated poor outcomes among animals with hyperglycemia during ischemia and reperfusion.[15] The current AHA guidelines recommend against tight glycemic control (defined as a target glucose range of 80–110 mg/dL) because of concerns for worsening neuronal metabolism.[8] Without much evidence, the AHA guidelines suggest moderate glycemic control targeting a glucose range of 144 to 180 mg/dL (8–10 mmol/L).[8] In a recent single-center observational study, glucose measurements over the first 48 hours of ICU admission were studied in 381 patients resuscitated from cardiac arrest.[15] Poor outcomes were associated with hyperglycemia and high glycemic variation.[15] Hyperglycemia during this period was independently associated with poor outcome.[15] These results suggest that glycemic management strategies for cardiac arrest survivors should avoid severe hyperglycemia and significant swings in blood glucose during the acute period.

TARGETED TEMPERATURE MANAGEMENT

Induced hypothermia has been used to prevent brain injury during cardioplegic surgery for decades. By extension, experimental animal data and small pilot studies suggested a benefit to induced hypothermia after resuscitation from cardiac arrest. The proposed neuroprotective mechanisms of induced hypothermia include reduction of the cerebral metabolic rate for oxygen, reduction of glutamate excitotoxicity, anti-inflammatory properties, and reduction of reactive oxygen species. The cerebral metabolic rate for oxygen decreases linearly with reduction in temperature, as demonstrated in literature from cardiac surgical procedures using hypothermic cardioplegia.[16] The decreased cerebral metabolic rate results in slower ATP consumption, improved glucose metabolism, and decreased acidosis.[17] In animal models of transient global ischemia, hypothermia prevents glutamate toxicity, thereby reducing downstream apoptotic pathways that contribute to secondary neuronal injury after cardiac arrest.[18] Other mechanisms of hypothermic neuroprotection include decreasing production of reactive oxygen species during reperfusion[19]; inhibiting inflammatory mediators, such as nuclear factor-kB[20]; and reducing inflammatory cell infiltration.[21] Hypothermia acts at multiple steps in the postischemia pathways of neuronal injury, making it an attractive therapy for neuroprotection after cardiac arrest.

Conversely, fever has been demonstrated to increase mortality and worsen neurologic outcomes in a variety of brain injuries, including stroke, subarachnoid hemorrhage, and traumatic brain injury.[22] In addition, animal models of cardiac arrest have demonstrated increased mortality, increased ischemic neuronal injury, and worse functional outcomes in animals that were hyperthermic after resuscitation compared with normothermic and hypothermic controls.[23,24]

HYPOTHERMIA AFTER CARDIAC ARREST CLINICAL TRIAL

Two studies published in 2002 demonstrated improved outcomes in patients treated with hypothermia after resuscitation from cardiac arrest.[25,26] The Hypothermia After Cardiac Arrest study randomized 275 patients with cardiac arrest caused by ventricular fibrillation or ventricular tachycardia to 24 hours of hypothermia using surface cooling with a target temperature of 32°C to 34°C or standard therapy.[25] The mean interval from ROSC to initiation of cooling was 105 minutes. The median interval was 8 hours to achieve the goal temperature. Hypothermia was then maintained for 24 hours, after which patients were passively rewarmed. The primary endpoint was a favorable outcome at 6 months as defined by Cerebral Performance Categories. At 6 months, 75 (55%) of 136 patients in the hypothermia group had a favorable outcome, compared with 54 (39%) of 137 patients in the standard treatment group.[25] In the standard treatment group, 76 (55%) of 138 patients were dead at 6 months, whereas 56 (41%) of 137 died in the induced hypothermia group.[25] Although the standard treatment group was considered a normothermic control group, some were actually hyperthermic during the first 2 days.

AUSTRALIAN HYPOTHERMIA CLINICAL TRIAL

The second study was an Australian single-center clinical trial evaluating the impact of induced hypothermia on discharge disposition and mortality.[26] This study randomized 77 patients who were resuscitated after ventricular fibrillation cardiac arrest to induced hypothermia (target temperature of 33°C) versus standard treatment. Surface cooling was initiated in the field. Hypothermia was maintained for 12 hours and patients were then passively rewarmed. In the hypothermia group, most patients achieved the target temperature within 6 hours. The primary outcome was measured by discharge disposition with a favorable outcome defined as discharge to home or a rehabilitation facility. In the hypothermia group, 21 (49%) of 43 patients had a favorable outcome, compared with 9 (26%) of 34 patients in the standard treatment group.[26]

Subsequent to these studies, a series of small clinical trials, cohort studies, and meta-analyses were published. In one retrospective study, survival and favorable outcome rates were compared at a single center before and after introduction of an induced hypothermia protocol for comatose cardiac arrest survivors.[27] In patients with cardiac arrest caused by ventricular fibrillation, in-hospital mortality was 46% in the hypothermia cohort compared with 61% in the prehypothermia cohort. Favorable outcomes were found in 35% of the hypothermia cohort compared with 15% of the prehypothermia cohort.[27] A recent Cochrane meta-analysis concluded that, based on pooled clinical trial results, induced hypothermia is effective at reducing mortality and improving neurologic outcomes after resuscitation from out-of-hospital cardiac arrest with an initial rhythm of ventricular tachycardia or ventricular fibrillation.[28] Because of the promising nature of these results, induced hypothermia was included in guidelines for the Internal Liaison Committee on Resuscitation[29] and the AHA[8] among other international groups.

TARGET TEMPERATURE MANAGEMENT CLINICAL TRIAL

Despite early adoption by many professional societies, there was persistent skepticism that induced hypothermia truly improves outcomes after cardiac arrest because the clinical trials enrolled only a small number of patients, used loosely defined outcome measures, and included patients with hyperthermia in the control group. For these reasons, a multicenter, randomized clinical trial was undertaken in 36 ICUs in Australia and Europe. The Target Temperature Management (TTM) trial enrolled adult patients with an initial Glasgow Coma Scale score less than 8 after resuscitation from out-of-hospital cardiac arrest irrespective of the initial rhythm.[30] Patients were randomized to target temperature of 33°C or 36°C using either surface or intravascular cooling for 28 hours followed by gradual rewarming. Patients in both arms were then maintained at normothermia (<37.5°C) until 72 hours from cardiac arrest. Outcomes were measured by 3-month mortality and functional outcome based on the cerebral performance category and modified Rankin Scale. The study enrolled 950 patients, which exceeded all of the prior hypothermia trials combined. The mortality rates were 48% in the 36°C group and 50% in the 33°C group and poor outcomes occurred in 52% of the 36°C group and 54% of the 33°C group.[30] There were no differences in outcome among any of the prespecified subgroups, including those with an initial rhythm of ventricular fibrillation. Although adverse events were similar between the two groups, hypokalemia occurred more frequently with the lower temperature target.[30]

The results of this large, well-designed clinical trial were surprising to many who had adopted induced hypothermia protocols. Although it is difficult to compare the results with earlier trials, the favorable outcome and mortality rates in both arms of the TTM trial were similar to the induced hypothermia group in prior clinical trials and observational studies. These results suggest a benefit to strict temperature control, whether it is 36°C or 33°C, during the first 72 hours as opposed to no temperature control. This benefit seems to derive from fever prevention, gradual rewarming, and induced normothermia during the first 3 days rather than hypothermia, per se. Beyond the first 72 hours, however, there does not seem to be a benefit for continued maintenance of strict normothermia.[31] In a retrospective multicenter clinical registry of 236 patients treated with induced hypothermia for cardiac arrest, 41% of patients developed hyperthermia after active temperature management was discontinued.[31] However, no difference was noted in mortality or favorable outcomes between patients who did or did not develop rebound hyperthermia. Only the patients who developed severe hyperthermia (>38.7°C) after rewarming had worse outcomes.[31]

SEDATION AND SHIVERING DURING TARGETED TEMPERATURE MANAGEMENT

Shivering has been demonstrated to impede achievement and maintenance of the target temperature and increase the metabolic rate.[32] The Bedside Shivering Assessment Scale was devised to create a standardized approach to shivering patients. Algorithms have been developed for escalating treatment of shivering in patients on targeted temperature management, including surface counterwarming, sedation, neuromuscular blockade, magnesium infusion, buspirone, and dexmedetomidine.[33] Although sedatives and paralytic agents are more effective at suppressing shivering, improving lactate clearance, and maintaining target temperature,[34] these agents obscure the neurologic examination and could mask awakening, progression to brain death, seizures, myoclonic jerks, and other important neurologic events. For this reason, after the target temperature is achieved, protocols typically suggest weaning sedatives and paralytics in favor of buspirone, magnesium, and dexmedetomidine.[33] Development of shivering during targeted temperature management is an important prognostic sign, because patients who are able to be cooled without shivering often have severe brain injuries involving hypothalamic control of body temperature. In one study, cardiac arrest patients who did not develop shivering during induced hypothermia had favorable outcomes 36% of the time compared with 60% in the group that developed shivering.[35]

NEUROMONITORING AFTER CARDIAC ARREST: CLINICAL EXAMINATION

Most cardiac arrest patients remain comatose during the initial evaluation in the emergency department.[8] During this period, the prognosis for neurologic recovery is usually unclear and providers need to make decisions regarding aggressiveness of care including PCI and targeted temperature management in rapid fashion. The initial clinical examination is the first step of neuromonitoring after resuscitation from cardiac arrest. Patients who remain comatose (Glasgow Coma Scale <8) may be appropriate for targeted temperature management, whereas those with early recovery of consciousness (purposeful movements, attending and tracking, following commands, or verbalizing) have not been included in clinical trials.[25,26] Conversely, patients with clinical signs of brain death after ROSC are unlikely to benefit from targeted temperature management, PCI, or other aggressive measures. After admission, serial bedside neurologic assessment is important for recognition of signs of early recovery of consciousness, progression to brain death, intracranial hypertension or cerebral herniation, postanoxic myoclonus, and seizures. All of these findings provide important prognostic information and inform changes in clinical management. During the initial ICU management, bedside neurologic testing should be performed every 1 to 2 hours.[8] Sedation and neuromuscular blockade should be minimized to facilitate the neurologic examination.

ICP Monitoring

Because global, transient anoxia-ischemia from cardiac arrest results in selective neuronal injury, even patients with severe brain injury after cardiac arrest usually do not develop significant mass effect from cytotoxic edema. Cardiac arrest survivors typically develop bland neuronal loss without significant cerebral edema, intracranial hypertension, or cerebral herniation.[36] In the small number of studies that report ICP and multimodality monitoring from comatose cardiac arrest survivors, the ICP was only rarely elevated.[36] In patients who develop severe cytotoxic cerebral edema leading to intracranial hypertension and cerebral herniation, medical management with corticosteroids, osmotic agents, and hyperventilation is usually ineffective. For this reason, placement of ICP monitors is rarely undertaken.

Electroencephalogram Monitoring and Seizure Detection

Electroencephalogram (EEG) is commonly ordered in comatose cardiac arrest survivors for prognosis and to detect nonconvulsive status epilepticus (NCSE) or occult seizures in patients requiring neuromuscular blockade for targeted temperature management. NCSE may produce subtle clinical signs, such as unexplained tachycardia, gaze deviation or nystagmus, tachypnea, abnormal posturing, or bruxism.[37] Because these signs may also be present in anoxic-ischemic brain injury, EEG is often needed to exclude seizures. If EEG recording is undertaken to evaluate a specific movement (eg, myoclonic jerks), a standard recording may be sufficient to determine if they represent seizures.[38] If an EEG is ordered to exclude NCSE, longer recordings (24–72 hours) may be needed.[39] When continuous EEG monitoring was undertaken in cardiac arrest survivors treated with hypothermia, NCSE was identified in 12%, most of which began within 12 hours of resuscitation.[40] The significance of detecting NCSE after cardiac arrest is unclear, however, because the prognosis is poor whether or not these postarrest seizures are treated.[40,41] A recent study comparing intermittent with continuous EEG in comatose cardiac arrest survivors with induced hypothermia found a 94% concordance rate for detection of epileptiform discharges, suggesting that continuous EEG monitoring may be unnecessary for most patients.[42]

Distinguishing NCSE from other EEG patterns, such as periodic epileptiform discharges and burst-suppression, can be challenging. This is especially true in post–cardiac arrest patients, in whom periodic EEG patterns are common. Determining which EEG patterns *cause* brain injury and which are a *marker* of existing brain injury is difficult.[43] There is high interobserver variability in EEG diagnosis of seizures in comatose patients.[44] For this reason, criteria have been proposed for defining electrographic seizures in NCSE.[44,45] This definition requires at least one of three primary criteria: (1) repetitive generalized or focal spikes, sharp waves, spike-and-wave, or sharp-and-slow complexes at greater than or equal to 3 Hz; (2) repetitive generalized or focal spikes, sharp waves, spike-and-wave, or sharp-and-slow complexes at a frequency of less than 3 Hz and the secondary criterion; or (3) sequential rhythmic, periodic, or quasiperiodic waves greater than or equal to 1 Hz and unequivocal evolution in frequency (incrementing and decrementing over time), morphology, or location and the secondary criterion. The secondary criterion is clinical improvement or emergence of normal, organized background EEG activity in response to benzodiazepine or other anticonvulsant drug administration.[45,46] More recently, there has been growing interest in separating classical NCSE, which typically occurs in awake but encephalopathic patients, from NCSE in coma.[47] To what extent the EEG phenomenon detected (1) is the cause of coma, (2) is treatable, or (3) contributes to worsening brain injury remain controversial.

PROGNOSTICATION AFTER CARDIAC ARREST: CLINICAL EXAMINATION

The American Academy of Neurology (AAN) issued a practice parameter for prognostication after cardiac arrest in 2006 (**Fig. 2**).[48] The resulting prognostic algorithm relies on bedside neurologic examination, electrophysiologic testing with EEG and somatosensory evoked potentials (SSEP), and cerebrospinal fluid (CSF) neuron-specific enolase (NSE) concentration. Complete absence of brainstem reflexes on the first day after ROSC, myoclonic status epilepticus on the first day, absence of pupillary light and corneal reflexes and/or absent motor responses other than extensor posturing after 72 hours, and bilateral absence of cortical N20 potentials on SSEP after 24 hours were

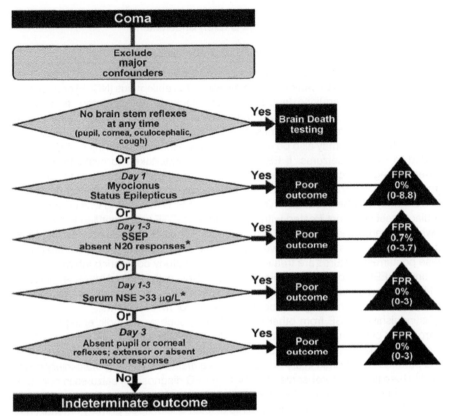

Fig. 2. Prognostic algorithm for comatose cardiac arrest survivors from the 2006 American Academy of Neurology Practice Parameter. * These test results may not be available on a timely basis. Serum NSE testing may not be sufficiently standardized. (*From* Wijdicks EF, Hijdra A, Young GB, et al. Practice parameter: prediction of outcome in comatose survivors after cardiopulmonary resuscitation (an evidence-based review). Neurology 2006;67:203–10; with permission.)

all considered highly specific markers of poor prognosis.[48] Poor prognosis was considered no improvement beyond persistent vegetative state. Although CSF NSE greater than 33 mg/dL was also included in the algorithm, subsequent studies have questioned its prognostic accuracy. Myoclonic status epilepticus is characterized by generalized, nonrhythmic, symmetric myoclonic jerks primarily involving the face and trunk that typically increase with stimulation.[48] These movements are generally described as agonal brain activity reflective of a severe, underlying brain injury rather than true epileptic seizures. Treatment of myoclonic status epilepticus with anticonvulsant medications is typically unsuccessful and has not been demonstrated to improve outcomes.[48]

Utility of SSEP in Prognostication

Standard SSEP testing after cardiac arrest uses scalp electrodes to assesses the brain's response to electrical stimulation of the median nerve at the wrist. The latency of conduction is normally 20 milliseconds to the primary sensory cortex. In global anoxic-ischemic brain injury, the primary cortical responses (N20) may be delayed or lost, reflecting loss of neural conduction from the brainstem or thalamus to cortex (**Fig. 3**). For prognostic

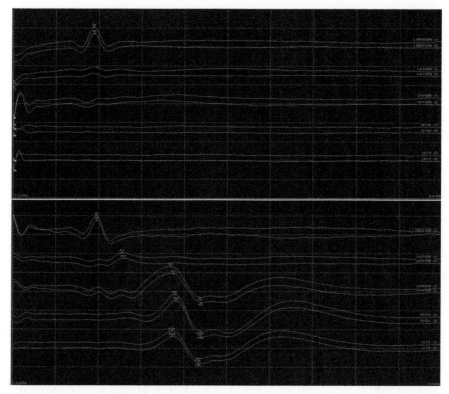

Fig. 3. Median nerve SSEP showing absent cortical N20 potential in a comatose cardiac arrest patient with poor prognosis (*top*) and present N20 potential in a cardiac arrest patient with favorable outcome (*bottom*).

purposes, SSEP should be performed 1 to 3 days after resuscitation from cardiac arrest.[48] Studies performed too early may result in a falsely pessimistic prognosis. After 24 hours, the persistent bilateral absence of cortical N20 potentials on median nerve SSEP studies has nearly 100% specificity for poor outcome in comatose cardiac arrest survivors with a false-positive rate of 0.7% (range, 0%–3.7%).[48] Although some authors have assessed the prognostic value of SSEP for determining which patients will have good neurologic recovery, no reliably specific marker has been identified at this point. Most patients with preserved N20 potentials still go on to have poor neurologic outcomes.[48]

Utility of EEG in Prognostication

EEG has also been extensively studied as a prognostic marker after cardiac arrest, but the ability to perform meta-analyses on the resulting data has been confounded by the variety of grading schemes used in individual studies. Most studies describe a series of malignant EEG patterns after cardiac arrest, including generalized EEG suppression, burst-suppression, alpha- or theta-coma, and NCSE patterns.[48] Burst-suppression is defined by alternating periods of generalized suppression interrupted by periods of generalized, high-voltage bursts (**Fig. 4**). Alpha- and theta-coma refer to patterns of unwavering, generalized alpha (8–12 Hz) or theta (4–7 Hz) activity that is present in all leads and has no variability in response to external stimulation. EEG patterns evolve during the first 24 hours after cardiac arrest. If EEG is performed early

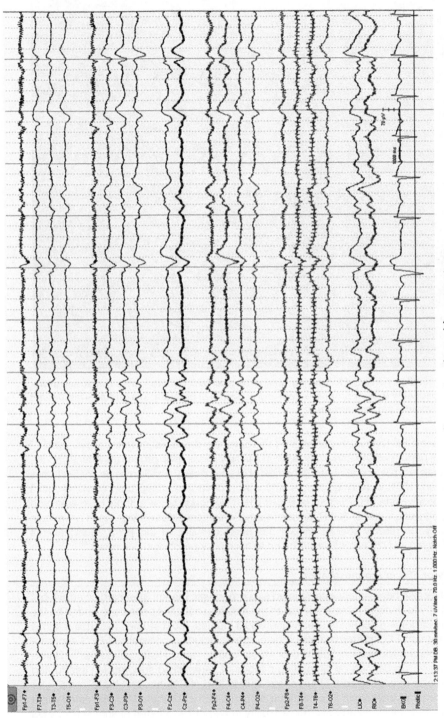

Fig. 4. EEG showing periodic suppression in a comatose cardiac arrest patient with poor outcome.

enough, most patients progress from electrocerebral silence through a period of burst-suppression before regaining continuous, reactive EEG patterns.[49] EEG is also heavily influenced by use of sedative agents. In the AAN consensus statement, the malignant patterns of EEG activity were strongly associated with poor outcomes after cardiac arrest but they had an unacceptably high false-positive rate of 3% (range, 0.9%–11%) and were not included in the final prognostic algorithm.[48] In a recent small series of cardiac arrest survivors treated with hypothermia, the presence of subjectively determined EEG reactivity was noted in 19 of 19 survivors, 14 of whom went on to have favorable neurologic outcomes, and only 3 of 15 nonsurvivors.[50] In another recent study, recovery of continuous EEG activity within 12 hours of resuscitation was strongly associated with good neurologic outcomes.[49]

Utility of Brain Imaging in Prognostication

The AAN practice parameter did not support the prognostic value of brain imaging with computed tomography (CT) or magnetic resonance imaging (MRI) in comatose cardiac arrest survivors.[48] The relative insensitivity of routine structural brain imaging sequences to detect brain injury from cardiac arrests reflects the pathophysiology of transient global hypoxia-ischemia, which causes selective neuronal injury while sparing the nonneuronal brain architecture. For this reason, even very severe neuronal loss results in radiographically bland brain injury during the acute period. A structurally normal brain CT or MRI has poor specificity for neurologic recovery in a comatose patient after resuscitation from cardiac arrest.[48] Recent studies have demonstrated greater prognostic accuracy using standardized methods to measure loss of distinction between gray matter and white matter indicating severe, global cytotoxic edema.[51] This method relies on measurement of Hounsfield units of gray matter and white matter in the putamen and internal capsule for calculation of the gray-white matter ratio (GWR) (**Fig. 5**). Although this method still needs to be validated,

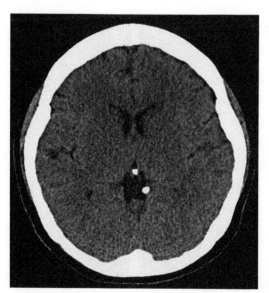

Fig. 5. Noncontrast head CT showing loss of distinction between gray matter and white matter in the basal ganglia and internal capsule, typical of cytotoxic edema from cardiac arrest.

abnormal GWR in CT performed 1 to 7 days after cardiac arrest was associated with poor prognosis with 100% specificity and 44% sensitivity in one study.[51]

Advanced MRI sequences are also being studied for prognostication after cardiac arrest. Diffusion-weighted imaging and apparent diffusion coefficient (ADC) maps are in widespread clinical use for stroke imaging. Although these sequences are qualitative, ADC can also be quantified and lower values reflect cerebral infarction. One study found that the percentage of brain volume with decreased ADC values was predictive of neurologic outcomes at 3 to 6 months.[52] Diffusion tensor imaging takes advantage of directional diffusion of protons to measure the integrity of subcortical white matter tracts based on fractional anisotropy values. In a prospective study of 57 comatose patients resuscitated from cardiac arrest, reduced fractional anisotropy demonstrated high specificity and sensitivity for predicting poor outcomes at 1 year.[53] Functional MRI (fMRI) studies changes in brain perfusion as a marker for regional activation. Using resting state fMRI, a default mode network has been identified that includes the anterior and posterior cingulate, precuneus, and temporal-parietal junction. The default mode network represents resting state brain activity and disruption of connectivity within this network has been found in chronic disorders of consciousness, anesthesia-induced unconsciousness, and coma.[54] Two recent small studies have demonstrated disruption of default mode network connectivity in patients with poor outcomes after cardiac arrest and preserved connectivity in patients who awoke after cardiac arrest (**Fig. 6**).[55,56] Despite promising results, further validation of ADC, diffusion tensor imaging, and resting-state fMRI sequences is required before they can be used for prognostication in routine clinical practice.

EFFECT OF INDUCED HYPOTHERMIA ON PROGNOSTIC MARKERS

The AAN practice parameter on prognostication after cardiac arrest was published before widespread use of induced hypothermia and all of the studies evaluated by

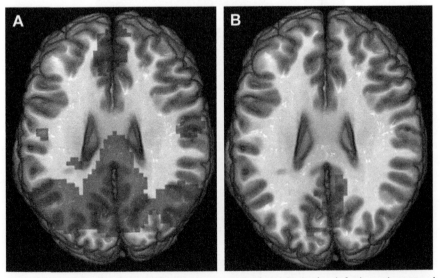

Fig. 6. Resting-state functional MRI showing preserved activity in the default mode network in cardiac arrest patients with favorable outcome (*A*) and disrupted default mode network activity in those with poor outcomes (*B*).

the authors were conducted before the hypothermia era. Because of the expected benefits of induced hypothermia, there was uncertainty that the prognostic accuracy of standard tests would be maintained among cardiac arrest patients treated with hypothermia.[48] In the last few years, several studies have re-evaluated the prognostic tests reviewed in the AAN practice parameter in cardiac arrest survivors treated with induced hypothermia. Because hypothermia slows peripheral conduction of electrical stimuli, SSEP performed during induced hypothermia must be interpreted with caution. For this reason, SSEP testing is more accurate after patients are rewarmed to normal body temperature. A few small series have determined that the bilateral absence of N20 potentials remains a highly specific marker of poor outcome whether or not patients were treated with hypothermia.[57] A recent meta-analysis of cardiac arrest patients treated with induced hypothermia supported the high specificity of bilateral absence of cortical N20 potentials for predicting poor outcomes.[58] The CSF NSE cut points cited in the AAN practice parameter are not reliable in patients treated with induced hypothermia and several studies have now documented patients with favorable neurologic recovery despite very high CSF NSE levels after being treated with induced hypothermia.[59]

Time to awakening, defined by purposeful movements and command following, may be delayed in patients treated with induced hypothermia. This delay may occur because a higher dose of sedative medications is needed in patients who are cooled, because clearance of sedatives is delayed at cooler body temperature, or because cooling actually alters the natural history of awakening after cardiac arrest. The prognostic accuracy of the motor examination, in particular, has been called into question in patients treated with hypothermia. Motor response no better than extensor posturing may no longer be a reliable indicator of poor outcome.[59] Several case series have investigated whether cooling impacts the time to awakening, with conflicting results. One single-center study found that no purposeful motor response beyond 72 hours continued to be highly specific for poor outcomes in patients treated with induced hypothermia.[60] Another multicenter study found that, among patients with favorable neurologic outcomes at discharge, the mean time to awakening was 2.8 days with an interquartile range of 2 to 4.5 days and some outliers with favorable outcomes despite awakening that was delayed beyond 7 days.[61] A recent meta-analysis of cardiac arrest patients treated with induced hypothermia concluded that, at 72 hours, the absence of purposeful motor responses had an excessively high false-positive rate of 0.21.[58] For this reason, many authors have recommended caution on rendering a final prognosis based solely on the motor examination at 72 hours in the absence of other negative prognostic indicators. Although a few case reports have appeared of hypothermia-treated patients with favorable neurologic outcomes despite myoclonus during the first 24 hours,[62] persistent myoclonic status epilepticus still seems to be highly specific to poor outcomes regardless of treatment with hypothermia. Similarly, the prognostic value of absent pupillary reflex does not seem to be affected by hypothermia.[58]

SUMMARY

Brain-directed therapies and prognostication in comatose patients resuscitated from cardiac arrest remains complex. Although recent studies have shown that survival and functional recovery after cardiac arrest have modestly improved with advances in critical care, outcomes still remain poor in most patients. The resources required for PCI, specialized critical care, targeted temperature management, multispecialty consultation, and prognostic testing are substantial. The results of the recent TTM study cast doubt on the efficacy of induced hypothermia and the accuracy of prognostic testing may be hindered by hypothermia. At this point, prognostic testing is directed toward late identification of patients who are destined to have poor outcomes. By the time this testing is complete (perhaps as late as 7 days if the provider is relying on the motor examination after induced hypothermia) significant resources have already been expended. Future work should focus on early identification of patients who are likely to benefit from aggressive care and early reliable markers that a patient is nonsalvageable. The clinical examination and electrophysiologic testing for prognosis are problematic during the acute period, especially with targeted temperature management. Many patients who ultimately have poor outcomes do not have highly specific markers, such as nonreactive pupils or bilateral absence of cortical N20 potentials. Most patients currently fall into an indeterminate prognostic category. Although standard clinical imaging has not been validated for prognosis, recent quantitative studies of GWR using CT and MRI ADC values suggest a role for imaging criteria in future early stratification of cardiac arrest survivors.

REFERENCES

1. Go AS, Mozaffarian D, Roger VL, et al. Heart disease and stroke statistics – 2013 update, a report from the American Heart Association. Circulation 2013; 127:6–245.
2. Arawwawala D, Brett SJ. Clinical review: beyond immediate survival from resuscitation – long-term outcome considerations after cardiac arrest. Crit Care 2007; 11:235–52.
3. Chalkias A, Xanthos T. Post-cardiac arrest brain injury: pathophysiology and treatment. J Neurol Sci 2012;315:1–8.
4. Hinduja A, Gupta H, Yang JD, et al. Hypoxic ischemic brain injury following in hospital cardiac arrest – lessons from autopsy. J Forensic Leg Med 2014;23:84–6.
5. Fujioka M, Okuchi K, Sakaki T, et al. Specific changes in human brain following reperfusion after cardiac arrest. Stroke 1994;25:2091–5.
6. Nolan JP, Neumar RW, Adrie C, et al. Post-cardiac arrest syndrome: epidemiology, pathophysiology, treatment, and prognostication. Resuscitation 2008; 79:350–79.
7. Horstmann A, Frisch S, Jentzsch RT, et al. Resuscitating the heart but losing the brain: brain atrophy in the aftermath of cardiac arrest. Neurology 2010;74:306–12.
8. Peberdy MA, Callaway CW, Neumar RW, et al. Post-cardiac arrest care: 2010 American Heart Association guidelines for cardiopulmonary resuscitation and emergency cardiovascular care. Circulation 2010;122:S768–86.
9. Larsen JM, Ravkilde J. Acute coronary angiography in patients resuscitated from out-of-hospital cardiac arrest – a systematic review and meta-analysis. Resuscitation 2012;83:1427–33.
10. Sideris G, Voicu S, Yannopoulos D, et al. Favourable 5-year postdischarge survival of comatose patients resuscitated from out-of-hospital cardiac arrest, managed with immediate coronary angiogram on admission. Eur Heart J Acute Cardiovasc Care 2014;3(2):183–91.
11. Kilgannon JH, Jones AE, Shapiro NI, et al. Association between arterial hyperoxia following resuscitation from cardiac arrest and in-hospital mortality. JAMA 2010;303:2165–71.
12. Vaahersalo J, Bendel S, Reinikainen M, et al. Arterial blood gas tensions after resuscitation from out-of-hospital cardiac arrest: associations with long-term neurological outcome. Crit Care Med 2014;42(6):1463–70.

13. del Castillo J, López-Herce J, Matamoros M, et al. Hyperoxia, hypocapnia and hypercapnia as outcome factors after cardiac arrest in children. Resuscitation 2012;83:1456–61.
14. Trzeciak S, Jones AE, Kilgannon JH, et al. Significance of arterial hypotension after resuscitation from cardiac arrest. Crit Care Med 2009;37:2895–903.
15. Daviaud F, Dumas F, Demars N, et al. Blood glucose level and outcome after cardiac arrest: insights from a large registry in the hypothermia era. Intensive Care Med 2014;40(6):855–62.
16. McCullough JN, Zhang N, Reich DL, et al. Cerebral metabolic suppression during hypothermic circulatory arrest in humans. Ann Thorac Surg 1999;67:1895–9.
17. Laptook AR, Corbett RJ, Burns D, et al. Neonatal ischemic neuroprotection by modest hypothermia is associated with attenuated brain acidosis. Stroke 1995; 26:1240–6.
18. Busto R, Globus MY, Dietrich WD, et al. Effect of mild hypothermia on ischemia-induced release of neurotransmitters and free fatty acids in rat brain. Stroke 1989;20:904–10.
19. Globus MY, Busto R, Lin B, et al. Detection of free radical activity during transient global ischemia and recirculation: effects of intraischemic brain temperature modulation. J Neurochem 1995;65:1250–6.
20. Han HS, Karabiyikoglu M, Kelly S, et al. Mild hypothermia inhibits nuclear factor-κB translocation in experimental stroke. J Cereb Blood Flow Metab 2003;23: 589–98.
21. Kumar K, Evans AT. Effect of hypothermia on microglial reaction in ischemic brain. Neuroreport 1997;8:947–50.
22. Greer DM, Funk SE, Reavan NL, et al. Impact of fever on outcome in patients with stroke and neurologic injury: a comprehensive meta-analysis. Stroke 2008;39:3029–35.
23. Jia X, Koenig MA, Venkatraman A, et al. Post-cardiac arrest temperature manipulation alters early EEG bursting in rats. Resuscitation 2008;78:367–73.
24. Jia X, Koenig MA, Nickl R, et al. Early electrophysiologic markers predict functional outcome associated with temperature manipulation after cardiac arrest in rats. Crit Care Med 2008;36:1909–16.
25. The Hypothermia after Cardiac Arrest Study Group. Mild therapeutic hypothermia to improve the neurologic outcome after cardiac arrest. N Engl J Med 2002; 346:549–56.
26. Bernard SA, Gray TW, Buist MD, et al. Treatment of comatose survivors of out-of-hospital cardiac arrest with induced hypothermia. N Engl J Med 2002;346:557–63.
27. Don CW, Longstreth WT, Maynard C, et al. Active surface cooling protocol to induce mild therapeutic hypothermia after out-of-hospital cardiac arrest: a retrospective before-and-after comparison in a single hospital. Crit Care Med 2009; 37:3062–9.
28. Arrich J, Holzer M, Havel C, et al. Hypothermia for neuroprotection in adults after cardiopulmonary resuscitation. Cochrane Database Syst Rev 2012;(9):CD004128.
29. Nolan JP, Morley PT, VandenHoek TL, et al. Therapeutic hypothermia after cardiac arrest: an advisory statement by the advanced life support task force of the International Liaison Committee on Resuscitation. Circulation 2003;108:118–21.
30. Nielsen N, Wettersley J, Cronberg T, et al. Targeted temperature management at 33°C versus 36°C after cardiac arrest. N Engl J Med 2013;369:2197–206.
31. Leary M, Grossestreuer AV, Iannacone S, et al. Pyrexia and neurological outcomes after therapeutic hypothermia for cardiac arrest. Resuscitation 2013; 84:1056–61.

32. Badjatia N, Strongilis E, Gordon E, et al. Metabolic impact of shivering during therapeutic temperature modulation: the bedside shivering assessment scale. Stroke 2008;39:3242–7.

33. Choi HA, Ko SB, Presciutti M, et al. Prevention of shivering during therapeutic temperature modulation: the Columbia anti-shivering protocol. Neurocrit Care 2011;14:389–94.

34. Salciccioli JD, Cocchi MN, Rittenberger JC, et al. Continuous neuromuscular blockade is associated with decreased mortality in post-cardiac arrest patients. Resuscitation 2013;84:1728–33.

35. Nair SU, Lundbye JB. The occurrence of shivering in cardiac arrest survivors undergoing therapeutic hypothermia is associated with a good neurologic outcome. Resuscitation 2013;84:626–9.

36. Nordmark J, Rubertsson S, Mörtberg E, et al. Intracerebral monitoring in comatose patients treated with hypothermia after cardiac arrest. ActaAnaesthesiol Scand 2009;53:289–98.

37. Friedman D, Claassen J, Hirsch LJ. Continuous electroencephalogram monitoring in the intensive care unit. Anesth Analg 2009;109:506–23.

38. Scozzafava J, Hussain MS, Brindley PG, et al. The role of the standard 20 minute EEG recording in the comatose patient. J Clin Neurosci 2010;17:64–8.

39. Claassen J, Mayer SA, Kowalski RG, et al. Detection of electrographic seizures with continuous EEG monitoring in critically ill patients. Neurology 2004;62: 1743–8.

40. Rittenberger JC, Popescu A, Brenner RP, et al. Frequency and timing of nonconvulsive status epilepticus in comatose post-cardiac arrest subjects treated with hypothermia. Neurocrit Care 2012;16:114–22.

41. Crepeau AZ, Rabinstein AA, Fugate JE, et al. Continuous EEG in therapeutic hypothermia after cardiac arrest, prognostic and clinical value. Neurology 2013; 80:339–44.

42. Alvarez V, Sierra-Marcos A, Oddo M, et al. Yield of intermittent versus continuous EEG in comatose survivors of cardiac arrest treated with hypothermia. Crit Care 2013;17:R190.

43. Bauer G, Trinka E. Nonconvulsive status epilepticus and coma. Epilepsia 2010; 51:177–90.

44. Ronner HE, Ponten SC, Stam CJ, et al. Inter-observer variability of the EEG diagnosis of seizures in comatose patients. Seizure 2009;18:257–63.

45. Chong DJ, Hirsch LJ. Which EEG patterns warrant treatment in the critically ill? Reviewing the evidence for treatment of periodic epileptiform discharges and related patterns. J Clin Neurophysiol 2005;22:79–91.

46. Seidel S, Aull-Watschinger S, Pataraia E. The yield of routing electroencephalography in the detection of incidental nonconvulsive status epilepticus – a prospective study. Clin Neurophysiol 2012;123:459–62.

47. Fernandez-Torre JL, Rebollo M, Gutierrez A, et al. Nonconvulsive status epilepticus in adults: electroclinical differences between proper and comatose forms. Clin Neurophysiol 2012;123:244–51.

48. Wijdicks EF, Hijdra A, Young GB, et al. Practice parameter: prediction of outcome in comatose survivors after cardiopulmonary resuscitation (an evidence-based review). Neurology 2006;67:203–10.

49. Cloostermans MC, van Meulen FB, Eertman CJ, et al. Continuous electroencephalography monitoring for early prediction of neurological outcome in post-anoxic patients after cardiac arrest: a prospective cohort study. Crit Care Med 2012;40:2867–75.

50. Rossetti AO, Urbano LA, Delodder F, et al. Prognostic value of continuous EEG monitoring during therapeutic hypothermia after cardiac arrest. Crit Care 2010; 14:173–81.

51. Gentsch A, Storm C, Leithner C, et al. Outcome prediction after cardiac arrest: a simplified method for determination of gray-white matter ratio in cranial computed tomography. Clin Neuroradiol 2014. [Epub ahead of print].

52. Wijman CA, Miynash M, Caulfield AF, et al. Prognostic value of brain diffusion weighted imaging after cardiac arrest. Ann Neurol 2009;65:394–402.

53. Luyt CE, Galanaud D, Perlbarg V, et al. Diffusion tensor imaging to predict long-term outcome after cardiac arrest: a bicentric pilot study. Anesthesiology 2012; 117(6):1311–21.

54. Vanhaudenhuyse A, Noirhomme Q, Tshibanda LJ, et al. Default network connectivity reflects the level of consciousness in non-communicative brain damaged patients. Brain 2010;133:161–71.

55. Norton L, Hutchison RM, Young GB, et al. Disruptions of functional connectivity in the default mode network of comatose patients. Neurology 2012;78:175–81.

56. Koenig MA, Holt JL, Ernst T, et al. MRI default mode connectivity is associated with functional outcome after cardiopulmonary arrest. Neurocrit Care 2014; 20(3):348–57.

57. Rothstein TL. Therapeutic hypothermia and reliability of somatosensory evoked potentials in predicting outcome after cardiopulmonary arrest. Neurocrit Care 2012;17:146–9.

58. Kamps MJ, Horn J, Oddo M, et al. Prognostication of neurologic outcome in cardiac arrest patients after mild therapeutic hypothermia: a meta-analysis of the current literature. Intensive Care Med 2013;39:1671–82.

59. Oddo M, Rossetti AO. Predicting neurological outcome after cardiac arrest. Curr Opin Crit Care 2011;17:254–9.

60. Fugate JE, Wijdicks EF, White RD, et al. Does therapeutic hypothermia affect time to awakening in cardiac arrest survivors? Neurology 2011;77:1346–50.

61. Grossestreuer AV, Abella BS, Leary M, et al. Time to awakening and neurological outcome in hypothermia-treated cardiac arrest patients. Resuscitation 2013;84: 1741–6.

62. Lucas JM, Cocchi MN, Salciccioli J, et al. Neurologic recovery after therapeutic hypothermia in patients with post-cardiac arrest myoclonus. Resuscitation 2012; 83:265–9.

Neuromuscular Complications of Critical Illness

Jules Osias, MD, MPH*, Edward Manno, MD

KEYWORDS

- Critical illness polyneuropathy • Critical illness myopathy
- Acute quadriplegic myopathy • Sepsis • Neuromuscular disorders

KEY POINTS

- Critical illness neuropathy and myopathy are neuromuscular complications of sepsis or are iatrogenic complications of treatments required in the intensive care setting.
- A combination of neuromuscular complications can occur in one patient.
- The severity of CIP/CIM depends on the length of ICU stay, severity of illness, and definitive diagnosis.
- Recovery depends on the degree of peripheral nerve axonal involvement.

BACKGROUND

Generalized weakness of limb and respiratory muscles in intensive care unit (ICU) patients is a long recognized phenomenon. Neuromuscular complications of critical illness are usually discovered in the patient that has difficulty in weaning from mechanical ventilation that cannot be explained by pulmonary or cardiac compromise.[1] Critical illness polyneuropathy (CIP) and critical illness myopathy (CIM) are the most common entities identified as the cause of neuromuscular weakness in the ICU.[1–3] In 1984, Bolton and colleagues[4] described a polyneuropathy that developed after sepsis and multiorgan failure. Later a myopathy initially linked to steroids and neuromuscular blocking agents (NMBA) was identified.

The association between sepsis and neuromuscular weakness has been known for more than 50 years. In 1955, Erbsloh[5] observed a polyneuropathy that developed in a patient after a prolonged coma. Mertens,[6] in 1961, described "coma-polyneuropathies" in patients who developed hypovolemic shock. Similarly, Bischoff and

Disclosures: None.
Neurological Institute, Cleveland Clinic Foundation, 9500 Euclid Avenue, Cleveland, OH 44195, USA
* Corresponding author.
E-mail address: osiasj@ccf.org

colleagues[7] in 1977 observed four patients develop a severe polyneuropathy after sepsis that they originally attributed to the use of gentamicin.

Charles Bolton, however, provided the most thorough analysis of this phenomenon in the early 1980s. In 1981, Bolton and colleagues[8] described five ICU patients who had difficulty weaning from the ventilator and severe limb weakness. Electrophysiologic studies revealed a primary axonal degeneration of motor and sensory fibers. At the time, possible etiologies including nutritional deficiencies, heavy metal toxicity, antibiotic use, collagen vascular disease, or spinal cord ischemia were ruled out. Therefore, it was suggested that sepsis itself was the underlying cause of the documented neuromuscular weakness.[1]

By 1983, a total of 19 cases of polyneuropathies were prospectively identified and studied through electrophysiologic testing by Bolton.[1] The term "critical illness polyneuropathy" was used to identify this neuropathy because it was clearly associated with sepsis and multiorgan failure. The neuropathy was similarly associated with the encephalopathy being described in patients with sepsis. In their study, 70% of patients with sepsis and multiorgan failure were affected by this polyneuropathy based on electrodiagnostic studies.[4]

APPROACH TO ACUTE NEUROMUSCULAR WEAKNESS IN THE ICU

The approach to a patient who is found to have weakness in the ICU should include a thorough history and general physical and neurologic assessment. The clinical examination may be limited by sedation and/or an encephalopathy. Despite this difficulty, the history, timing, and pattern of weakness must be assessed to differentiate the cause. For example, a distal bilateral motor involvement after a recent infectious illness suggests Guillain-Barré syndrome (GBS). Hyporeflexic quadriparesis after awakening from trauma suggests an acute spinal cord injury. Unilateral limb involvement could be explained by a plexopathy, whereas weakness confined to a single nerve distribution strongly points toward a compression neuropathy.

GBS and myasthenia gravis are neuromuscular disorders directly admitted to the ICU primarily for progressive respiratory weakness, yet critical illness can exacerbate these diseases. Identifying the neuropathy or myopathy associated with critical illness as the source of neuromuscular weakness is important because it may help to avoid performing unnecessary studies, such as imaging of the brain.

Many patients with neuromuscular weakness in the ICU are identified because of failure to wean from mechanical ventilation. Up to 30% of ICU patients may experience difficulty in weaning off the ventilator.[9] Common causes for inability to wean from mechanical ventilation should be ruled out first and include cardiac, pulmonary, and chest wall dysfunction. Neurologic causes account for the other etiologies of failure to wean.[2] In one study, central neurologic causes for failure to wean including stroke and depressed mental status accounted for 26% of all cases. Peripheral neurologic sources accounted for another 17%.[9] CIP was usually the source of peripheral nervous system failure, whereas other peripheral nerve sources (ie, unilateral phrenic neuropathy, defects in neuromuscular transmission, and myopathy) accounted for the remainder. The number of cases identified as peripheral nerve sources of ventilator failure increased with increased use of electrophysiologic studies.

Electrodiagnostic studies are important in the evaluation of patients with neuromuscular weakness and allow for localization of the injury to the motor nerve, neuromuscular junction, or muscle. They may, however, be difficult to perform and interpret in the ICU setting and usually require more than 3 weeks of symptoms to arrive at a diagnosis.[10]

Electrophysiologic studies including phrenic nerve conduction evaluation, despite its technical difficulties, can be performed in the ICU to establish the cause of neuromuscular weakness. Subclavian vein catheters or chest injuries may limit phrenic nerve studies. Diaphragmatic electromyography (EMG) can be performed in addition to phrenic nerve conduction velocities to assess for a myopathy. Repetitive nerve stimulation can also be added to exclude neuromuscular transmission, such as myasthenia or Lambert-Eaton syndrome, as the cause of respiratory failure.[10]

CIP

CIP is one of the most common neuromuscular complications of critical illness occurring in 25% to 50% of patients admitted to the ICU with the systemic inflammatory response syndrome (SIRS) or sepsis.[11,12] SIRS occurs in 20% to 50% of patients in ICUs; thus, CIP can be a significant contributor to morbidity. These percentages increase up to 47% to 70% if electrodiagnostic evidence of an axonal sensorimotor polyneuropathy is used to detect CIP.[12–16]

CIP is usually preceded by a septic encephalopathy followed by difficulty in weaning from mechanical ventilation. The severity and duration of illness and hyperglycemia and poor nutritional status may also contribute to the neuropathy.[15]

Because clinical examinations are usually limited in these patients, signs of polyneuropathy may not be apparent in about half of the patients.[17] In CIP the motor nerves are disproportionally affected earlier and to a greater degree than the sensory nerves. On examination, a patient may grimace to painful peripheral stimulation, but be unable to withdraw the limb. The sensory nerves are involved later in the course of the disease and to a lesser degree than motor involvement. Deep tendon reflexes are preserved until late in the disease process.[1] Muscle atrophy is a sign of advanced disease and may represent muscle that is functionally disconnected from its nerve or a secondary CIM. Sensory testing may show evidence of distal loss of pain, temperature, and vibration sense. Cerebrospinal fluid is usually normal, although mildly elevated protein levels may occur.

Electrophysiology

Electrodiagnostic studies are important in the diagnosis of CIP. These studies should include motor and sensory nerve conduction and EMG of the upper and lower limbs. For a diagnosis of CIP, findings should be consistent with primary, axonal degeneration.[4,8,10] A reduction in compound muscle action potential and sensory nerve action potential amplitudes should be observed. Moreover, a study documenting phrenic nerve involvement establishes CIP as the cause of failure to wean off the ventilator.[10]

Performance and interpretation of electrodiagnostic studies in the ICU may be difficult. Cycle artifacts from other electronic devices are common, especially on sensory nerve conduction studies (NCS) and needle EMG. Therefore, one should be cautious to minimize interference by turning off unnecessary equipment. It should be noted, however, that fibrillation potentials and other abnormal spontaneous discharges can be heard even when they cannot be seen.[10]

Other issues that may complicate the performance and interpretation of electrodiagnostic studies include limb edema and decreased extremity body temperature. Patients in the ICU may often be peripherally vasoconstricted and cool to touch and require a warming blanket before testing. Edema at recording sites may be responsible for low-amplitude sensory nerve action potentials and therefore adjustments should be made to account for this.[10]

Differential Diagnosis

To diagnose CIP, a patient must be critically ill, show difficulty in weaning off the ventilator after such causes as heart and lung disease are excluded, demonstrate limb weakness on clinical examination, and have electrophysiologic evidence of axonal motor and sensory polyneuropathy.[1] Other neuromuscular process in the ICU should also be ruled out before a diagnosis of CIP. The most difficult differentiation with CIP is the motor nerve variant of GBS. Electrodiagnostically, these entities are very similar. The differential rests in the history and clinical course. The motor variant of GBS occurs abruptly and typically occurs before ICU admission. Antiganglioside M1 antibodies can be found in a significant percentage of patients, although this finding is not specific to GBS. CIP develops slowly and progressively during sepsis. A pure motor neuropathy in association with NMBAs has also been reported. Although it is possible that worsening neuropathy in the ICU might be caused by GBS, if electrodiagnostic studies are consistent with axonal degeneration, CIP is the more likely diagnosis.

Neuromuscular weakness can result from transient but prolonged neuromuscular blockade in patients receiving high doses and infusions of neuromuscular blockers. This is especially seen in the setting of induced hypothermia where metabolism and clearance is slowed, or in renal failure patients who are receiving vecuronium, which has an active metabolite, 3-desacetylvecuronium, that is renally cleared. Repetitive nerve stimulation, however, can easily allow one to differentiate between a neuromuscular transmission problem and neuromuscular blockade.

Prolonged recumbence, direct trauma, and hemorrhagic compression can explain mononeuropathies and plexopathies, which may coexist with CIP or CIM.

Pathophysiology

Several observations about CIP have provided speculation to its cause.[15–18] First, the neuropathy occurs in the setting of sepsis suggesting some intrinsic factor that is released during sepsis that must be participating in this process. Second, the neuropathy occurs in a length-dependent fashion from distal to proximal. Third, CIP tends to be more severe with longer length of stay in ICU, elevated serum glucose, and decreasing serum albumin. Finally, energy expenditure studies of peripheral nerves during sepsis reveal decreased metabolism.

These observations have led authors to speculate that CIP may be caused by a defect in axonal transport of nutrients. Nutrients in the cell body are transported through the axon to distal portions of the nerve through a process that requires significant energy expenditure. Sepsis releases various interleukins and cytokines that may affect mitochondrial use of oxygen and, thus, the energy needed for nutrient transport.

Similarly, the microcirculation to peripheral nerve is likely impaired by sepsis and elevated glucose levels.[18] Because vessels supplying the peripheral nerves lack autoregulation, they are specifically vulnerable to the effects of sepsis. Cytokines that are released during sepsis increase permeability of the microvasculature. Hyperglycemia and hypoalbuminemia, in turn, can induce edema leading to ischemia of distal portions of the peripheral nerves. Moreover, critically ill patients with neuromuscular disorders have been found to have enhanced expression of E-selectin in endothelium of epineurial and endoneurial vessels, which suggests endothelial cell activation likely caused by sepsis.[19] Such findings support the idea that axonal degeneration is the major pathologic feature of CIP.

Treatment

CIP is associated with SIRS and sepsis. Therefore any treatment that minimizes the degree and length of time the patient is septic has a significant improvement on the degree of CIP.[1,17,20] It follows that avoidance of SIRS and sepsis is important in preventing CIP. Although a critical care practitioner cannot prevent SIRS before admission to the ICU, while in the ICU, factors that increase the risks for developing sepsis should be minimized and early aggressive treatment of sepsis should be initiated as soon as possible. Management of CIP should include treatment of sepsis and multiorgan failure, avoidance of steroids and NMBAs because those can lead to CIM, and early mobilization with physiotherapy and rehabilitation.[12,21–23]

Studies have shown improvement of CIP with glucose control in critically ill patients. Van den Berghe and colleagues[24] in 2001 showed that invasive insulin therapy leads to a 44% reduction in CIP. Thus, although the debate about tight glucose control continues in the critical care literature, more aggressive control of glucose levels seems to significantly decrease the degree of neuropathy that develops during sepsis.

Attempts at treating CIP with intravenous immunoglobulin have not shown improvement.[25] Muscle strengthening exercises can be considered if there has been significant reinnervation of respiratory muscles. However, if the cause of respiratory weakness is not CIP, muscle strengthening exercises may not be of value.

Prognosis

Recovery from CIP depends on the severity of illness. The distance over which axonal regeneration must occur is associated with the degree and timing of recovery.[4] More severe illness may be correlated with a longer distance over which axonal regeneration must occur. Neurophysiologic and clinical evidence of a polyneuropathy may remain for up to 5 years after discharge from the ICU.[1] Patients with more severe illness may actually remain quadriplegic if axonal transection has occurred.[26]

CIM

CIM is a collective term encompassing all myopathies that present after admission to an ICU.[1,27–30] The term itself does not necessarily imply an underlying pathology because many forms of the disease exist, including critical care myopathy, acute necrotizing myopathy of intensive care, thick filament myopathy, CIM, acute corticosteroid myopathy, acute myopathy in severe asthma, acute hydrocortisone myopathy, and acute corticosteroid and pancuronium-associated myopathy. To be considered CIM, weakness must ensue after the onset of critical illness.[1]

There are fewer prospective studies of CIM when compared with CIP. Major risk factors include steroid use and severity of illness. In one prospective study, 7% of patients who underwent liver transplantation developed severe weakness caused by CIM.[31] The reported incidence of CIM in patients with status asthmaticus and chronic obstructive pulmonary disease is approximately 35%.[32]

Risk factors for the development of CIM include disease severity, SIRS, use of catecholamines, and elevated levels of insulin growth factor binding protein 1.[1,2,10,33] A definite diagnosis of CIM requires the first five of the following features[1,30]:

- Sensory nerve action potentials amplitudes greater than 80% of the lower limit of normal
- Needle EMG with short duration, low-amplitude motor unit action potentials with or without normal recruitment, with or without fibrillation potentials
- Absence of a decremental response on repetitive nerve stimulation

- Histopathology showing myosin loss
- Elevated creatinine kinase (CK)
- Muscle inexcitability

An acute quadriplegic myopathy (AQM) was first described in 1977 in a patient with asthma who was treated with corticosteroids and NMBAs.[34] The classic patient with AQM is one with asthma who is intubated for an acute asthma exacerbation and treated with steroids and paralytics. The quadraparetic/plegic myopathy is discovered after sedation and paralysis are withdrawn. The examination reveals an awake and alert quadriplegic patient with intact cranial nerves. Cervical cord injury is typically evaluated and ruled out as a source of the quadriplegia. The diagnosis is made with EMG and muscle biopsy. The original description reported myosin filament loss (see later). AQM, however, can also be detected in patients with sepsis who are not treated with steroids and paralytics.[35]

Neuromuscular blockade can lead to the development of a myopathy and masquerade as a myopathy. NMBAs used to facilitate mechanical ventilation can accumulate in the setting of hepatic and/or renal failure.[36] As a result, failure of these organs may lead to a prolonged effect of NMBAs after the drug has been discontinued. Repetitive nerve stimulation correctly identifies this defect in neuromuscular transmission by showing a decremental response in compound muscle action potential. Studies should be repeated 7 to 10 days after cessation of paralytics unless blockade is so severe that no motor response can be recorded.[17]

Many studies have shown that NMBAs, such as pancuronium or vecuronium, when used with corticosteroids can cause either a pure axonal motor neuropathy or a primary myopathy.[32,37–40] In these settings NMBAs are used for prolonged periods of time (usually days or weeks). Difficulty in weaning from the ventilator and limb paralysis may be observed after the drugs are discontinued and EMG/NCS reveal severe axonal degeneration in the motor nerves.[1] Needle EMG may show fibrillations and positive sharp waves, whereas muscle biopsy may show different degrees of muscle necrosis, atrophy, and thick filament myosin loss.[38]

This type of neuromuscular weakness is thought to be a result of a combination of functional denervation as a result of neuromuscular blockade and the direct effect of steroids on muscle.[1] The diagnosis can become even more complicated because a severe CIP can functionally de-enervate the distal musculature, subsequently putting the affected muscles at risk for developing CIM.

Although a functional or acquired denervation of the distal musculature may facilitate the development of a myopathy, it is not required, nor does it occur in all patients.[41] Many patients with sepsis develop a myopathy without being pharmacologically paralyzed.[35] The underlying mechanisms and pathology of these processes, however, are most likely different.

Thick Filament Myosin Loss

This syndrome usually occurs in severe asthma cases requiring ventilator support, high-dose steroid, and NMBAs. It can also be seen in post liver transplant patients who have received these medications.[31] Mild elevations in CK may be observed. Destruction of thick myosin filaments can often be detected on light microscopy but electron microscopy analysis is definitive. The mechanism of how this occurs in unclear; however, it has been noted that steroid receptors on myosin fibrils increase when muscle is disconnected from its innervation. There is no specific treatment of this syndrome. Recovery may also be more rapid than CIP.[1]

Rhabdomyolysis

Rhabdomyolysis occurs in critical illness. It is associated with severe hypophosphatemia. It presents with myalgia, weakness, and swelling. Severe muscle necrosis results in hyperkalemia and hypocalcemia caused by release of potassium and sequestration of calcium, which in turn can lead to life-threatening cardiac arrhythmias and renal failure.[27] Serum CK levels is elevated sometimes up to 10,000 IU/L.[1]

Needle EMG findings usually show infrequent fibrillation potentials and normal motor unit potentials, whereas motor and sensory NCS are usually normal.[42] Muscle biopsy may be normal or show myofiber necrosis without inflammation, myosin loss, or other specific features.[1] The mechanism of how this occurs is unclear.

Cachectic Myopathy

Starvation and malnutrition can also cause muscle weakness and wasting, as is the case in severe eating disorders, such as anorexia nervosa.[43] It accounts for significant wasting and weakness of muscle. EMG/NCS findings and CK levels are normal. Muscle biopsy may be normal or show type 2 fiber atrophy.[1] Cachectic myopathy is a diagnosis of exclusion.

Acute Necrotizing Myopathy

This syndrome is likely a variation of the acute rhabdomyolysis seen in critically ill patients.[44] It may be related to a secondary infectious agent of toxin.[45] It is characterized by myonecrosis with vacuolization and phagocytosis of muscle fibers. Although it was initially described in the context of steroid use in patients with asthma, it became clear by the 1990s that NMBAs were also associated with acute necrotizing myopathy and that the duration of muscular blockade is a prominent risk factor.[32] Serum CK levels are highly elevated and myoglobinuria is present. EMG/NCS studies show severe myopathy, and biopsies show widespread necrosis of muscle fibers.[46] The severity of illness may impede recovery of muscle strength.[26]

Pathophysiology

The role of steroids and NMBAs in CIM is not clearly understood. It is possible that NMBAs cause denervation, which may facilitate the toxic effect of other agents, such as steroids.[15] Animal studies show that denervation results in proliferation of steroid receptors on muscle membranes and that subsequent steroid use led to muscle thick filament loss and loss of muscle excitability.[47]

In CIM, muscle wasting, as evidenced by increased loss of urinary nitrogen, and protein catabolism are observed. Muscle biopsies show low glutamine levels, low protein/DNA levels, and high concentrations of extracellular water. The body's requirement for glutamine is likely not met during critical illness despite the relative influx of glutamine in muscle during illness. Glutamine, therefore, may be a "conditionally essential" amino acid during critical illness.[48]

Electrodiagnostic studies in CIM reveal muscle inexcitability. Animal model studies suggest that this inexcitability may be related to inactivation of sodium channels that subsequently adjusts the resting membrane potential of the muscle.[49] Upregulation of proteolytic pathways and apoptotic markers have similarly been observed. In 2002, Brealy and colleagues[50] found an association between antioxidant depletion and nitric oxide overproduction, with mitochondrial dysfunction, and decreased ATP concentrations, which leads to organ failure. Therefore, it is a reasonable speculation that related inhibition of complex I of the respiratory chain may be an important cause of depletion of muscle ATP and energy failure.

Treatment

Similar to CIP, aggressive treatment of sepsis will likely reduce the incidence of CIM. Because increased ICU length of stay is associated with severity of illness, measures that reduce duration in the ICU should be taken. Studies of anabolic hormones have not shown efficacy. No treatments have proved to be helpful to this point.[1]

The risk of developing CIM in association with corticosteroids and NMBA seems to increase after 24 to 48 hours of therapy.[51] Because there seems to be a relationship between steroids and NMBA administration and the development of CIM, the use of these agents should be limited as much as possible. Prolonged neuromuscular blockade should be avoided by scheduling frequent drug holidays with evidence of recovery from NMBAs, such as patient movement.[15]

SUMMARY

CIP and CIM or a combination of the two are common neuromuscular complications of sepsis and can be iatrogenic complications of treatments required in the ICU. Electrodiagnostic studies and muscle biopsy can help in the diagnosis and prognosis of neuromuscular weakness. Glycemic control, early mobilization, and judicious use of steroids and NMBAs are the primary approaches to reduce the incidence and severity of neuromuscular complications in ICU patients.

REFERENCES

1. Bolton CF. Neuromuscular manifestations of critical illness. Muscle Nerve 2005; 32:140–63.
2. Latronico N, Shehu I, Seghelini E. Neuromuscular sequelae of critical illness. Curr Opin Crit Care 2005;11:381–90.
3. Linos K, Foot C, Ziegenfuss M, et al. Critical illness weakness: common questions. Curr Anaesth Crit Care 2007;18:252–60.
4. Bolton CF, Gilbert JJ, Hahn AF, et al. Polyneuropathy in critically ill patients. J Neurol Neurosurg Psychiatr 1984;47:1223–31.
5. Erbsloh F. Polyneuritic pathological conditions in internal medicine. Munch Med Wochenschr 1955;97:753–6.
6. Mertens HG. Disseminated neuropathy following coma. On the differentiation of so-called toxic polyneuropathy. Nervenarzt 1961;32:71–9.
7. Bischoff A, Meier C, Roth F. Gentamicin neurotoxicity (polyneuropathy-encephalopathy). Schweiz Med Wochenschr 1977;107:3–8.
8. Bolton C, Brown J, Sibbald W. The electrophysiologic investigation of respiratory paralysis in critically ill patients. Neurology 1983;33:186.
9. Lemaire F. Difficult weaning. Intensive Care Med 1993;19:S69–73.
10. Lacomis D. Electrophysiology of neuromuscular disorders in critical illness. Muscle Nerve 2013;47:452–63.
11. Bolton CF, Young GB, Zochodne DW. The neurological complications of sepsis. Ann Neurol 1993;33:94.
12. Leijten FS, De Weerd AW, Poortvliet DC, et al. Critical illness polyneuropathy in multiple organ dysfunction syndrome and weaning from the ventilator. Intensive care Med 1996;22:856–61.
13. Khan J, Harrison TB, Rich MM. Mechanisms of neuromuscular dysfunction in critical illness. Crit Care Clin 2008;24(1):165.

14. Leijten FS, Harinck-de Weerd JE, Portvliet DC, et al. The role of polyneuropathy in motor convalescence after prolonged mechanical ventilation. JAMA 1995; 274:1221–5.

15. Pandit L, Agrawal A. Neuromuscular disorders in critical illness. Clin Neurol Neurosurg 2006;108:621–7.

16. Witt NJ, Zochodne DW, Bolton CF, et al. Peripheral nerve function in sepsis and multiple organ failure. Chest 1991;99:176–84.

17. Bird SJ, Rich MM. Neuromuscular complications of critical illness. Neurologist 2000;6:2–11.

18. Glauser MP, Zanetti G, Baumgartner JD, et al. Septic shock: pathogenesis. Lancet 1991;338:732–6.

19. Fenzi F, Latronico N, Refatti N, et al. Enhanced expression of E-selectin on the vascular endothelium of peripheral nerve in critically ill patients with neuromuscular disorders. Acta Neuropathol 2003;106:75–82.

20. Berek K, Margreiter J, Willeit J, et al. Polyneuropathies in critically ill patients: a prospective evaluation. Intensive Care Med 1996;22:849–55.

21. De Jonghe B, Sharshar T, Lefaucheur JP, et al. Paresis acquired in the intensive care unit: a prospective multicenter study. JAMA 2002;288:2859–67.

22. De Letter MA, Schmitz PI, Visser LH, et al. Risk factors for the development of polyneuropathy and myopathy in critically ill patients. Crit Care Med 2001;29: 2281–6.

23. Latronico N, Fenzi F, Recupero D, et al. Critical illness myopathy and neuropathy. Lancet 1996;347:1579–82.

24. Van den Berghe G, Wouters P, Weekers F, et al. Intensive insulin therapy in the critically ill patients. N Engl J Med 2001;345:1359–67.

25. Mohr M, Englisch L, Roth A, et al. Effects of early treatment with immunoglobulin on critical illness polyneuropathy following multiple organ failure and gramnegative sepsis. Intensive Care Med 1997;23:1144–9.

26. Zochodne DW, Thompson RT, Driedger AA, et al. Critical illness polyneuropathy. A complication of sepsis and multiple organ failure. Brain 1987;110:819–41.

27. Bird SJ. Myopathies and disorders of neuromuscular transmission. In: Brown W, Bolton C, Aminoff M, editors. Neuromuscular function and disease. Philadelphia: WB Saunders; 2002. p. 1507–20.

28. Eriksson LI. Acquired neuromuscular disorders in the critically ill patient. Seminars in Anesthesia, Perioperative Medicine and Pain 2002;21(2):135–9.

29. Hund E. Myopathy in critically ill patients. Crit Care Med 1999;27(11):2544–7.

30. Lacomis D, Zochodne DW, Bird SJ. Critical illness myopathy. Muscle Nerve 2000;23:1785–8.

31. Campellone JV, Lacomis D, Kramer DJ, et al. Acute myopathy after live transplantation. Neurology 1998;50:46–53.

32. Douglass JA, Tuxen DV, Horne M, et al. Myopathy in severe asthma. Am Rev Respir Dis 1992;146:517–9.

33. Bolton CF, Latronico N. Critical illness polyneuropathy and myopathy: a major cause of muscle weakness and paralysis. Lancet Neurol 2011;10:931–41.

34. MacFarlane IA, Rosenthal FD. Severe myopathy after status asthmaticus. Lancet 1977;2:615.

35. Rich MM, Bird SJ, Raps EC, et al. Direct muscle stimulation in acute quadriplegic myopathy. Muscle Nerve 1997;20:665–73.

36. Segredo V, Caldwell JE, Matthay MA, et al. Persistent paralysis in critically ill patients after long-term administration of vecuronium. N Engl J Med 1992;327: 524–5.

37. Barohn RJ, Jackson CE, Rogers SJ, et al. Prolonged paralysis due to nondepolarizing neuromuscular blocking agents and corticosteroids. Muscle Nerve 1994; 17:647–54.
38. Danon MJ, Carpenter S. Myopathy with thick filament (myosin) loss following prolonged paralysis with vecuronium during steroid treatment. Muscle Nerve 1991;14:1131–9.
39. Faragher MW, Day BJ, Dennett X. Critical care myopathy: an electrophysiological and histological study. Muscle Nerve 1996;19:516–8.
40. Giostra E, Magistris MR, Pizzolato G, et al. Neuromuscular disorder in intensive care unit patients treated with pancuronium bromide. Occurrence in a cluster group of seven patients and two sporadic cases, with electrophysiologic and histologic examination. Chest 1994;106:210–20.
41. Hoke A, Rewcastle NB, Zochodne DW. Acute quadriplegic myopathy unrelated to steroids or paralyzing agents: quantitative EMG studies. Can J Neurol Sci 1999;26:325–9.
42. Al-Jaberi M, Katirji B. The value of EMG in rhabdomyolysis. Muscle Nerve 1995; 18:1043.
43. McLoughlin DM, Spargo E, Wassif WS, et al. Structural and functional changes in skeletal muscle in anorexia nervosa. Acta Neuropathol 1998;95:632–40.
44. Zochodne DW, Ramsay DA, Saly V, et al. Acute necrotizing myopathy of intensive care: electrophysiological studies. Muscle Nerve 1994;17:285–92.
45. Ramsay DA, Zochodne DW, Robertson DM, et al. A syndrome of acute severe muscle necrosis in intensive care unit patients. J Neuropathol Exp Neurol 1993; 52:387–98.
46. Helliwell TR, Coakley JH, Wagenmakers AJ, et al. Necrotizing myopathy in critically-ill patients. J Pathol 1991;164:307–14.
47. Rich MM, Pinter MJ, Kraner SD, et al. Loss of electrical excitability in an animal model of acute quadriplegic myopathy. Ann Neurol 1998;43:171–9.
48. Burnham EL, Moss M, Ziegler TR. Myopathies in critical illness: characterization and nutritional aspects. Nutrition 2005;135:1818S–23S.
49. Rich MM, Teener JW, Raps EC, et al. Muscle is electrically inexcitable in acute quadriplegic myopathy. Neurology 1996;46:731–6.
50. Brealy D, Brand M, Hargreaves I, et al. Association between mitochondrial dysfunction and severity and outcome of septic shock. Lancet 2002;360:219–23.
51. Leatherman JW, Fluegel WL, David WS, et al. Muscle weakness in mechanically ventilated patients with severe asthma. Am J Respir Crit Care Med 1996;153: 1686–90.

Adverse Neurologic Effects of Medications Commonly Used in the Intensive Care Unit

(®) CrossMark

Stacy A. Voils, PharmD, MS, BCPS[a], Theresa Human, PharmD, BCPS[b], Gretchen M. Brophy, PharmD, BCPS[c],*

KEYWORDS

- Adverse effects • Neurologic complications • Drug interactions • Critical care
- Neurocritical care

KEY POINTS

- A detailed medication history should be performed and maintenance medications which are associated with potential withdrawal or rebound effects should be restarted if the benefit outweighs the risk.
- Numerous medications commonly used in the intensive care unit (ICU) have been associated with seizures.
- Benzodiazepines, opioids, corticosteroids, and histamine receptor antagonists have been associated with neurologic side effects, including delirium.
- Sedative, analgesic, and cardiovascular medications have been associated with increased intracranial pressure in patients in the ICU.
- Drug fever may occur at any time after initiation of the offending agent, but commonly occurs between 7 to 10 days.

INTRODUCTION

Polypharmacy is typical in most critically ill patients, which increases the risk for adverse effects and drug interactions. Furthermore, many patients have multiple comorbidities which require continuation of maintenance medications that may complicate their intensive care unit (ICU) course. Therefore, the pharmacotherapy of each patient must be evaluated to avoid adverse neurologic effects of commonly used ICU medications.

Disclosures: None.
[a] Department of Pharmacotherapy and Translational Research, University of Florida College of Pharmacy, 1225 Center Drive, HPNP Building, Room 3315, PO Box 100486, Gainesville, FL 32610-0486, USA; [b] Barnes-Jewish Hospital, Washington University in St. Louis, St. Louis, MO 63110, USA; [c] Departments of Pharmacotherapy & Outcomes Science and Neurosurgery, Medical College of Virginia Campus, Virginia Commonwealth University, 410 North, 12th Street, Richmond, VA 23298-0533, USA
* Corresponding author.
E-mail address: gbrophy@vcu.edu

Crit Care Clin 30 (2014) 795–811
http://dx.doi.org/10.1016/j.ccc.2014.06.009
0749-0704/14/$ – see front matter © 2014 Elsevier Inc. All rights reserved.

criticalcare.theclinics.com

This article focuses on medications commonly used in critically ill patients that can cause unwanted neurologic effects, and provides clinical pearls to avoid adverse drug events and drug interactions.

NEUROLOGIC COMPLICATIONS FROM MEDICATION DISCONTINUATION

Critically ill patients often require multiple medications for treatment of their acute injury. However, before starting these therapies and evaluating the potential for adverse effects and drug-drug interactions, it should be recognized that several of the patient's home medications may cause complications on abrupt discontinuation. Therefore, a detailed medication history should be performed and maintenance medications which are associated with potential withdrawal or rebound effects should be restarted if the benefit outweighs the risk. The pharmacokinetic characteristics of the individual medication will provide information regarding when withdrawal effects may begin to be observed (ie, approximately 3–5 times the half-life of the medication), and should be used to determine the window for reinitiation of therapy. **Table 1** lists

Table 1
Intensive care unit medications commonly associated with withdrawal symptoms

Drug Category	Withdrawal/Rebound Complications	Recommendations for Reinitiation of Therapy (Time After Last Dose)
Baclofen[8]	Delirium, hallucinations, agitation, muscle rigidity, hyperthermia, tachycardia, seizures	<12–24 h
Benzodiazepines[9–11]	Seizures, restlessness, anxiety, sleep disturbances, tremors, hallucinations, sweating	<48–72 h for short-acting agents; <4–7 d for long-acting agents
β-blockers[12,13]	Hypertension, tachycardia, myocardial ischemia	<24–48 h
Caffeine and Fioricet (40 mg caffeine/dose)[14,15]	Rebound headaches, decreased alertness	<12–24 h
Clonidine[16–19]	Hypertensive crisis, tachycardia, tremor, headache, anxiety, agitation	<18–36 h
Opioids[9–11]	Agitation, diaphoresis, nausea, vomiting, arthralgias, hypertension, tachycardia	<24–72 h
SSRIs[20,21]	Flu-like symptoms (nausea, vomiting, headache, lethargy), dizziness, paresthesias, tremors	<72 h (most common with shorter-acting SSRIs [eg, paroxetine > fluvoxamine > sertraline > fluoxetine])
Statins[4–7,22,23]	Cerebrovascular events, cardiovascular events	<24–48 h
Steroids (dosages ≥20 mg prednisone equivalents per day for ≥5 d or smaller doses for longer durations)[24]	Acute adrenal crisis, hypotension, fatigue, nausea, vomiting, abdominal pain, fever	Variable

Abbreviation: SSRI, selective serotonin reuptake inhibitor.

medications for which abrupt discontinuation should be avoided and their potential withdrawal or rebound complications.

Patients can also experience withdrawal from substances of abuse, such as ethanol and nicotine.[1] Symptoms of ethanol withdrawal can begin within 24 hours of the last drink and include hypertension, tachycardia, agitation, delirium, restlessness, tremors, seizures, hallucinations, and anxiety/pain; without treatment, these can be fatal.[2,3] Nicotine withdrawal symptoms often include agitation and restlessness, but nicotine replacement therapy is not required and can induce other neurologic adverse effects, such as headache, dizziness, and nervousness.

In patients with cerebrovascular or cardiovascular injuries, the withdrawal of statin therapy has been associated with poor outcomes from a rebound effect. This rebound effect has been attributed to the loss of the statins' pleiotropic effects, which include improved vascular function, antithrombotic activity, and anti-inflammation effects. Statin withdrawal has been shown to increase the risk of subarachnoid hemorrhage (SAH) in patients by more than 60% compared with those not taking a statin, and more than double the risk compared with patients who do not stop taking their statin. The largest effect is seen in those who also recently discontinued their hypertensive medication.[4] An increased risk of vasospasm in SAH patients in whom statins were discontinued has also been reported.[5] Poor outcomes have also been reported in patients who have sustained a stroke, with a 3-fold increase in mortality within the first year after an acute ischemic stroke in those who discontinued statin therapy compared with those who continued treatment, and almost a 20-fold increase in the risk of neurologic deterioration compared with patients who did not use statins.[6,7] Therefore, the benefits of restarting statin therapy on ICU admission and avoiding withdrawal rebound are clinically significant, and administration should not be interrupted.

DRUG-INDUCED SEIZURES

Seizures are associated with significant morbidity and mortality in critically ill patients, and range from convulsive status epilepticus, of which generalized tonic-clonic seizures are the most common, to the more insidious nonconvulsive status epilepticus. Risk factors for seizures in patients in the ICU include those related to the following underlying neurologic disorders[25]:

- Brain tumor
- Infection
- Head trauma
- History of seizures
- Stroke

Other risks for seizures may be related to the following complications seen in critical illness:

- Hypoxia
- Sepsis
- Drug withdrawal or overdose
- Electrolyte or endocrine disorders[26]
  - Sodium abnormalities
  - Hypocalcemia
  - Hypomagnesemia
  - Hypoglycemia

The presence of one or more of these coexisting risk factors may predispose patients in the ICU to seizures from the additive effect of drugs that lower the seizure threshold. However, the frequency of medication-induced seizures is unknown, owing to variability in reporting and difficulty in establishing causality, because patients in the ICU often have multiple risk factors for seizures.

Drugs Associated with Seizures

Anti-infective medications have frequently been implicated as a cause of drug-induced seizures. Penicillins and structurally related antibiotics (eg, cephalosporins, carbapenems, and monobactams) and fluoroquinolones are most commonly described in case reports and series as being associated with drug-induced seizures. Carbapenem antibiotics have the highest reported rates of seizures for any drug, with an incidence of 0.3% to 33.0%.[27] Seizures may occur less frequently with newer carbapenems (doripenem, meropenem, and ertapenem), although some trials reporting higher rates of imipenem-cilastatin–induced seizures included patients with other possible explanations for seizures.[28] The antituberculosis agent isoniazid has also been implicated in drug-induced seizures, mostly in cases of overdose; however, case reports describe seizures in patients receiving isoniazid at therapeutic doses.[29]

Psychotropic medications such as phenothiazines, selective serotonin reuptake inhibitors, tricyclic antidepressants, and bupropion have been associated with seizures. Chlorpromazine has the highest reported incidence of seizures among the phenothiazines appears to be dose-related, reportedly occurring more often in patients receiving greater than 1000 mg/d.[25,30] Selective serotonin receptor inhibitors have a lower incidence of seizures compared with bupropion and tricyclic antidepressants. The highest incidence of reported seizures among the antipsychotic class of medications is clozapine, with a cumulative risk of 10% in a group of 1418 patients treated for up to 3.8 years. Clozapine-related seizures also seem to be dose-related, occurring more frequently in patients receiving dosages of 300 mg/d or more.[30]

Analgesic medications have the potential to increase risk of seizures, especially when combined with certain other medications or when used in patients with renal dysfunction. Tramadol should not be used in patients who are receiving selective serotonin reuptake inhibitors, tricyclic antidepressants, monoamine oxidase inhibitors, and central nervous system depressant medications.[31,32] In addition, caution should be used when administering tramadol to patients with central nervous system disorders (eg, history of seizures, stroke, or traumatic brain injury). Dosages of tramadol should be limited to no more than 200 mg/d administered no more frequently than every 12 hours in patients with renal impairment.

Meperidine should be avoided for routine use in patients in the ICU, because one of its active metabolites (normeperidine) has been associated with seizures. This agent should be avoided especially in patients with renal dysfunction, because it is renally eliminated and has approximately 3 times the central nervous system effects of meperidine. In addition, use of meperidine within 14 days of monoamine oxidase inhibitors is contraindicated, because this may lead to serotonin syndrome and related seizures.[33]

Medications that have been implicated in drug-induced seizures are shown in **Table 2.**

Seizures related to drug overdose are relatively common; In patients admitted to the emergency department reports show that 6.1% of new-onset seizures and 9% of seizures in status epilepticus involve drug toxicity. Among calls to a California

Table 2
Medications that may induce seizures

Antibiotics	Antidepressants
Cefepime	Bupropion
Erythromycin	Tricyclic antidepressants
Imipenem	MAOIs
Isoniazid	SSRIs
Levofloxacin	Trazodone
Linezolid	Venlafaxine
Meropenem	Analgesics
Metronidazole	Alfentanil
Penicillins	Fentanyl
Pyrimethamine	Meperidine
Antivirals	Morphine
Acyclovir	NSAIDs
Foscarnet	Pentazocine
Ganciclovir	Propoxyphene
Antifungals	Tramadol
Amphotericin B	Hypoglycemics
Fluconazole	Insulin
Antineoplastics	Metformin
Busulfan	Immunosuppressant agents
Carmustine (BCNU)	Cyclosporine
Chlorambucil	Hydrocortisone
Cisplatin	Interferon-a
Cytarabine	Methylprednisolone
Methotrexate	Muromomab-CD3
Vinblastine	Sulfasalazine
Vincristine	Tacrolimus
Anesthetic agents	Pulmonary agents
Bupivacaine	Albuterol
Enflurane	Aminophylline
Etomidate	Terbutaline
Halothane	Theophylline
Isoflurane	Cardiovascular agents
Ketamine	Atropine
Lidocaine	Digoxin
Mepivacaine	Esmolol
Methohexital	Ephedrine
Procaine	Flecainide
Propofol	Oxytocin
Sevoflurane	Propranolol
Tetracaine	Miscellaneous agents
Psychoactive agents	Baclofen
Clozapine	Bromocriptine
Haloperidol	Desmopressin
Lithium	Flumazenil
	(*continued on next page*)

Table 2 (continued)	
Olanzapine	Levodopa
Risperidone	Methylphenidate
Phenothiazines	Metoclopramide
	Metrizamide
	Physostigmine

Abbreviations: BCNU, bis-chloronitrosourea; MAOI, monoamine oxidase inhibitor; NSAID, nonsteroidal anti-inflammatory agent; SSRI, selective serotonin reuptake inhibitor.

Data from Voils SA, Brophy GM. Drug-induced seizures. In: Papadopoulos J, editor. Drug-induced complications in the critically ill patients: a guide for recognition and treatment. Mount Prospect (IL): Society of Critical Care Medicine; 2012. p. 117; and Tesoro EP, Brophy GM. Pharmacologic management of seizures and status epilepticus in critically ill patients. J Pharm Pract 2010; 23(5):441–54.

poison control center in 2003, the most common medications associated with seizures were[34]

- Bupropion (23%)
- Diphenhydramine (8.3%)
- Tricyclic antidepressants (7.7%)
- Tramadol (7.5%)
- Amphetamines (6.9%)
- Isoniazid (5.9%)
- Venlafaxine (5.9%)

Among recreational drugs, the most common were

- Cocaine (5%)
- 3,4-methylenedioxymethamphetamine, or "ecstasy" (3%)

Mechanisms of Drug-Induced Seizures

Although the β-lactam ring alone is epileptogenic, structural differences among β-lactam and related antibiotics may be associated with convulsant activity (**Box 1**).[27,35,36]

The proposed mechanisms of drug-induced seizure activity for several medications are shown in **Table 3**.

In addition to inherent drug characteristics, other factors may lead to a predisposition for seizures,[27,32,37–39] such as high dosages and/or

- Renal impairment in patients receiving drugs with high renal clearance
- Low inherent drug binding to albumin or a relative increase in free drug fraction because of reduced levels of plasma proteins (including albumin) that commonly occur with uremia
- Preexisting central nervous system disorder
- History of epilepsy
- Electrolyte abnormalities
- Combination with other drugs that lower seizure threshold
- Rapidly titrated doses
- Drug interactions
- Drugs with active metabolites associated with seizures (eg, meperidine)
- Drug withdrawal (eg, alcohol, benzodiazepines, propofol, baclofen)

Box 1
Structural differences among antibiotics that may be associated with convulsant activity

- β-lactams
  - Addition of an amino group onto basic penicillin structure (decreased convulsant activity)
    - Ampicillin
    - Amoxicillin
  - Addition of a ureido group onto basic penicillin structure (decreased convulsant activity)
    - Piperacillin
- Cephalosporins
  - Addition of a heterocyclic ring at position 7 on the basic cephalosporin structure (no convulsant activity)
    - Cefoxitin
    - Cefuroxime
  - Addition of a tetrazole ring at position 7 on the basic cephalosporin structure (increased convulsant activity)
    - Cefazolin
  - Addition of a heterocyclic ring at position 3 and an aromatic nucleus at position 7 on the basic cephalosporin structure (moderately increased convulsant activity)
    - Ceftriaxone
    - Ceftazidime
    - Cefotetan
- Carbapenems
  - Increased basicity of the carbon-2 substitution on the carbapenem ring associated with greater affinity for the γ-aminobutyric acid (GABA) type A receptor complex
    - More basic (increased convulsant activity)
      - Imipenem
    - Less basic (decreased convulsant activity)
      - Meropenem
      - Ertapenem
- Fluoroquinolones
  - Piperazine ring substitutions at the 7 position on the parent fluoroquinolone molecule
    - Unsubstituted (increased convulsant activity)
      - Norfloxacin
      - Ciprofloxacin
    - Methyl substitution (decreased convulsant activity)
      - Ofloxacin
      - Levofloxacin

Table 3
Proposed mechanism of drug-induced seizures

Drug	Mechanisms
Anti-infectives	
Penicillins and structurally related drugs	Inhibits GABA binding to $GABA_A$ receptor Blocks $GABA_A$ chloride channel
Fluoroquinolones	Inhibit GABA binding to $GABA_A$ receptor
Isoniazid	Inhibits pyridoxine kinase, resulting in decreased GABA synthesis
Metronidazole	Leads to accumulation of hydroxy- and 1-acetic acid metabolite
Psychotropics	
Bupropion	Increases noradrenergic activity
Selective serotonin reuptake inhibitors	Decreases GABA transmission in the hippocampus
Tricyclic antidepressants	Inhibits GABA binding to $GABA_A$ receptor
Phenothiazines	Antagonizes postsynaptic, mesolimbic dopamine receptors in the brain
Miscellaneous	
Local anesthetics	Antagonizes Na+ channels
Meperidine	Leads to accumulation of normeperidine metabolite
Tramadol	Inhibits monoamine uptake
Theophylline	Antagonizes anticonvulsant effects of brain adenosine
Calcineurin inhibitors	Downregulates $GABA_A$ receptor activation

Abbreviations: GABA, γ-aminobutyric acid; $GABA_A$, γ-aminobutyric acid type A; Na, sodium.

From Voils SA, Brophy GM. Drug-induced seizures. In: Papadopoulos J, editor. Drug-induced complications in the critically ill patients: a guide for recognition and treatment. Mount Prospect (IL): Society of Critical Care Medicine; 2012. p. 119.

Clinical pharmacists should be consulted for assessment of drug interactions and appropriate dose adjustments in patients with renal impairment.

DRUG-INDUCED PSYCHOSIS/DELIRIUM

Delirium has been associated with higher mortality, an increase in hospital and ICU length of stay, prolonged mechanical ventilation, and progressive cognitive decline. However, in a recent survey, only 25% of hospital ICUs in the United States reported consistent screening for delirium with a validated assessment tool.[40] Several medications commonly used in patients in the ICU have been associated with delirium.

Sedation with dexmedetomidine has been associated with a lower incidence of delirium when compared with midazolam and lorazepam, although an overall lighter sedation achieved in the dexmedetomidine groups may have contributed to the positive results.[41,42] The relationship between opioid use and development of delirium in patients in the ICU is unclear and data are conflicting.[43]

Glucocorticoid medications have been associated with many psychiatric conditions, such as depression, psychosis, confusion, disorientation, akathisia, and sleep and memory deficits. The onset of symptoms may occur within a few days of initiation and generally within the first few weeks of therapy.[44,45] Risk factors for glucocorticoid-related neurologic side effects reportedly include a history of neuropsychiatric disorder,[46] an inconsistent association with gender,[46,47] and increasing age.[46,48]

Furthermore, dosages of prednisone or the equivalent of greater than 20 mg/d increase the incidence of glucocorticoid-associated psychiatric syndromes[49]:

- Less than 40 mg/d: 1.3%
- 41 to 80 mg: 4.6%
- Greater than 80 mg: 18.4%

One study showed that the use of corticosteroids in noncomatose patients with acute lung injury in the ICU was associated with transition to delirium. Patients diagnosed with delirium received median prednisone-equivalent dosages of 44 mg/d compared with 23 mg/d for those without delirium.[48]

Benzodiazepine and alcohol withdrawal are associated with the following neurologic symptoms in patients in the ICU, including individuals who are receiving benzodiazepine medications for sustained periods while hospitalized[43]:

- Seizures
- Anxiety
- Tremor
- Headache
- Hyperactive delirium

Histamine-2 receptor antagonists have been associated with the following central nervous system adverse effects[50]:

- Delirium
- Agitation
- Psychosis
- Confusion
- Disorientation
- Hallucinations
- Hostility

Characteristics of adverse effects related to histamine-2 receptor antagonists include[50]:

- Onset during the first 2 weeks of therapy
- Generally resolved within 3 to 7 days of discontinuation
- Common with cimetidine
- Associated with advanced age (>60 years)
- More common in patients in the ICU
- Unclear relationship of dose and organ function with adverse effects

DRUG-INDUCED INCREASED INTRACRANIAL PRESSURE

Several uncontrolled studies report on the propensity of drugs to increase intracranial pressure (ICP) in patients with severe neurologic injury. Much of the published literature has focused on sedative and analgesic medications since these are routinely administered to patients with intracranial hypertension.

A recent systematic review assessing patient outcomes, adverse events, ICP, and cerebral perfusion pressure in critically ill patients with severe traumatic brain injury who received various sedative medications reported the following findings[51]:

- Morphine, fentanyl, sufentanil, and alfentanil significantly increased ICP and decreased cerebral perfusion pressure (CPP) and mean arterial pressure (MAP) after administration of bolus doses. These changes were generally transient,

but CPP and MAP remained decreased for 24 hours in one study.[52] Opioid dosing regimens in the included studies were as follows:
- o Fentanyl, 2–10 mcg/kg
- o Morphine, 0.2 mg/kg
- o Sufentanil, 0.6–1 mcg/kg
- o Alfentanil, 100 mcg/kg
- Ketamine infusions at mean dosages of 82–95 mcg/kg/min combined with midazolam infusions did not increase ICP or decrease CPP.
- Of the 5 included studies that assessed clinical outcomes, no differences among sedatives were noted in mortality, neurologic outcome, ICU length of stay, or quality of sedation.

The review[51] did not include any patients who received the opioid remifentanil but this agent does not seem to increase ICP.[53–55]

Although data in patients with neurologic injuries are scarce, the effect of a depolarizing neuromuscular blockading agent (eg, succinylcholine) on cerebral hemodynamics is variable.[56,57] Fasciculations may be associated with increases in ICP; for this reason, nondepolarizing neuromuscular blockers are often used in conjunction with succinylcholine.[58,59]

Medications used for acute blood pressure management in patients in neurocritical care unit have been shown to have variable effects on ICP.

- Agents generally considered to increase ICP with unknown clinical significance:
  - o Nitroprusside.[60–62] One study found an association between nitroprusside and increased in-hospital mortality when compared with nicardipine after adjusting for baseline risk of mortality in patients with intracerebral hemorrhage.[63] The authors speculate that nitroprusside may have led to decreases in cerebral perfusion pressure and increased ischemia, but none of these cerebral hemodynamic values were reported in this study.
  - o Nitroglycerin[64–66]
  - o Hydralazine[67]
- Agents generally considered to have neutral effect on ICP:
  - o Nicardipine[68,69]
  - o Clevidipine[70]
  - o Labetalol[71,72]

DRUG-INDUCED FEVER

Drug-induced fever is characterized by a febrile response coinciding with the administration of a medication and occurring in the absence of an underlying condition that can cause fever, which is most commonly infection.[73,74] Drug-induced fevers are generally a diagnosis of exclusion and often overlooked during the initial fever workup.[75] Drug-induced fever is estimated to be responsible for 3% to 5% of the adverse reactions to medications, and significantly impacts patient care through increasing the length of stay and health care costs.[73,76,77]

Pathophysiologically, medications can cause fever through several mechanisms, with the median time between initiation of the offending agent and the onset of fever reported to be between 7 to 10 days, although fever may occur at any point during the course of therapy (**Table 4**).[74] Abnormal laboratory values and clinical findings may support the diagnosis of drug-induced fever, although they not always reliable because they are not present in all cases. Concurrent cutaneous manifestations, leukocytosis, and eosinophilia have been reported in up to 29%, 22%, and 22% of patients with drug fever, respectively.[76]

Table 4
Mechanisms of drug-induced fever and common offending agents

	Altered Thermoregulation	Anticholinergic	Serotonin Syndrome	Malignant Hyperthermia	Neuroleptic Malignant Syndrome	Hypersensitivity	Antimicrobials
Mechanism of drug-induced fever	Increased heat production	↓ heat loss through changes in sweat gland secretions	Excessive activation of postsynaptic serotonin receptors	↑ cytoplasmic calcium-inducing skeletal muscle contraction & ↑ cell metabolism resulting ↑ heat & lactate production	↓ CNS dopamine activity	Humoral or cellular immune activation	Possible hypersensitivity
Common offending agents	Thyroxine Cocaine MDMA Amphetamine Epinephrine	Atropine Antihistamines TCA phenothiazines Antiparkinson meds	SSRI SNRI Opiates Trazodone Buspirone Mirtazapine Linezolid Metoclopramide Ondansetron	Succinylcholine Inhaled anesthetics	Block dopamine receptors Antipsychotic (typical > atypical) Metoclopramide Droperidol Prochlorperazine Withdrawal of dopaminergic agents: L-dopa Amantadine Bromocriptine Ropinirole Pramipexole Pergolide	Anticonvulsant Phenytoin Carbamazepine Heparin Allopurinol Procainamide	β-lactams Piperacillin Cefotaxime Imipenem Sulfonamides Amphotericin

(continued on next page)

Table 4
(continued)

	Altered Thermoregulation	Anticholinergic	Serotonin Syndrome	Malignant Hyperthermia	Neuroleptic Malignant Syndrome	Hypersensitivity	Antimicrobials
Onset	Variable	Variable	Variable	Immediate to hours after exposure	Variable	Variable	1–5 wk depending on prior antibiotic exposure
Possible treatment	Sympatholytic (benzodiazepine)		Benzodiazepine Cyproheptadine	Dantrolene	Bromocriptine Dantrolene		
Clinical pearls		↑ risk in geriatric patients Drug-induced fever does not occur with all agents in each drug class listed Phenothiazine + anticholinergics together ↑ fever risk	Common in ICU when multiple agents are used	Supplemental oxygen important because oxygen depleted rapidly in acute MH Nondepolarizing NMB may be used in severe cases Avoid CCB with dantrolene	Symptoms may evolve over 24–72 h High risk with large doses of antipsychotics, rapid titration, or multiple agents	Initial fever from offending agent may take days to weeks but will occur within hours with rechallenge Temporal relationship to drug timing may be key in identifying	Concomitant eosinophilia (25%), rash (5%) ↑ risk in HIV positive patients May take days for fevers to resolve after discontinuation Patient seems more stable than fever curve would indicate

Abbreviations: ↓, decreased; ↑, increased; CCB, calcium channel blockers; CNS, central nervous system; MDMA, 3,4-methylenedioxy-N-methylamphetamine; MH, malignant hyperthermia; NMB, neuromuscular blockers; SNRI, serotonin-norepinephrine reuptake inhibitors; SSRI, selective serotonin reuptake inhibitors; TCA, tricyclic antidepressants.

Fever associated with anticonvulsant use (specifically phenytoin, carbamazepine, oxcarbazepine, valproic acid, phenobarbital, and lamotrigine) can progress to drug reaction with eosinophilia and systemic symptoms (DRESS) syndrome. This syndrome has a longer latency period compared with other drug reactions (2–6 weeks) and typically affects at least one organ, most commonly the lungs, kidneys, liver, or heart. However, encephalitis, meningitis, and polyneuritis have been reportedly associated with DRESS syndrome.[78]

Treatment

If appropriate, discontinuation of the most likely offending agent is recommended, although determining the most likely agent and finding a suitable therapeutic alternative can be challenging. Resolution of the fever generally occurs within 48 to 72 hours, although reports have been published of fevers continuing weeks after the offending agent was discontinued, most commonly in cases in which cutaneous manifestations are recognized or the elimination half-life is prolonged.[74,79]

Rechallenge

Rechallenge in patients with drug-induced fever must be approached with extreme caution and is often not recommended.[80] Rechallenge may be performed to confirm the diagnosis of drug-induced fever, but only after the risks and benefits of reintroducing the medication have been considered.

SUMMARY

Adverse drug effects often complicate the care of critically ill patients. Therefore, a detailed medication history should be performed and maintenance medications which are associated with potential withdrawal or rebound effects should be restarted if the benefit outweighs the risk. Assessment of risk factors and, when appropriate, implementation of alternative therapy may prevent neurocognitive adverse effects of medications. Numerous medications commonly used in patients in the ICU have been associated with seizures. Although the incidence of drug-related seizures in patients in the ICU is unknown, the cause is considered multifactorial and patient-specific factors must be considered to minimize risk. Benzodiazepines, opioids, corticosteroids, and histamine receptor antagonists have been associated with neurologic side effects, including delirium. Sedative, analgesic, and cardiovascular medications have been associated with increased ICP in patients in the ICU. Studies addressing clinical outcomes in patients with neurologic disorders receiving sedatives have not shown a relationship between increased ICP and mortality, neurologic outcome, ICU length of stay, or quality of sedation. Drug-induced fever may occur at any time after initiation of the offending agent, but commonly occurs between 7 to 10 days, and should be considered in all febrile cases when the cause of the fever cannot be elucidated. Early diagnosis of drug-induced fever may reduce unnecessary diagnostic interventions and medications, such as antibiotics. Discontinuation of the most likely offending agent is recommended, if appropriate, and rechallenge should generally be avoided.

REFERENCES

1. Awissi DK, Lebrun G, Fagnan M, et al. Alcohol, nicotine, and iatrogenic withdrawals in the ICU. Crit Care Med 2013;41(9 Suppl 1):S57–68.
2. Awissi DK, Lebrun G, Coursin DB, et al. Alcohol withdrawal and delirium tremens in the critically ill: a systematic review and commentary. Intensive Care Med 2013;39(1):16–30.

3. McKeon A, Frye MA, Delanty N. The alcohol withdrawal syndrome. J Neurol Neurosurg Psychiatry 2008;79(8):854–62.
4. Risselada R, Straatman H, van Kooten F, et al. Withdrawal of statins and risk of subarachnoid hemorrhage. Stroke 2009;40(8):2887–92.
5. Singhal AB, Topcuoglu MA, Dorer DJ, et al. SSRI and statin use increases the risk for vasospasm after subarachnoid hemorrhage. Neurology 2005;64(6):1008–13.
6. Colivicchi F, Bassi A, Santini M, et al. Discontinuation of statin therapy and clinical outcome after ischemic stroke. Stroke 2007;38(10):2652–7.
7. Blanco M, Nombela F, Castellanos M, et al. Statin treatment withdrawal in ischemic stroke: a controlled randomized study. Neurology 2007;69(9):904–10.
8. Ross JC, Cook AM, Stewart GL, et al. Acute intrathecal baclofen withdrawal: a brief review of treatment options. Neurocrit Care 2011;14(1):103–8.
9. Birchley G. Opioid and benzodiazepine withdrawal syndromes in the paediatric intensive care unit: a review of recent literature. Nurs Crit Care 2009;14(1):26–37.
10. Cammarano WB, Pittet JF, Weitz S, et al. Acute withdrawal syndrome related to the administration of analgesic and sedative medications in adult intensive care unit patients. Crit Care Med 1998;26(4):676–84.
11. Devlin JW, Mallow-Corbett S, Riker RR. Adverse drug events associated with the use of analgesics, sedatives, and antipsychotics in the intensive care unit. Crit Care Med 2010;38(Suppl 6):S231–43.
12. Frishman WH. Beta-adrenergic blocker withdrawal. Am J Cardiol 1987;59(13): 26F–32F.
13. Mehta JL, Lopez LM. Rebound hypertension following abrupt cessation of clonidine and metoprolol. Treatment with labetalol. Arch Intern Med 1987;147(2): 389–90.
14. Rogers PJ, Heatherley SV, Mullings EL, et al. Faster but not smarter: effects of caffeine and caffeine withdrawal on alertness and performance. Psychopharmacology (Berl) 2013;226(2):229–40.
15. Rogers PJ, Smith JE. Caffeine, mood and cognition. In: Benton D, editor. Oxford (England): Woodhead; 2011. p. 251–71.
16. Hansson L, Hunyor SN, Julius S, et al. Blood pressure crisis following withdrawal of clonidine (Catapres, Catapresan), with special reference to arterial and urinary catecholamine levels, and suggestions for acute management. Am Heart J 1973;85(5):605–10.
17. Simic J, Kishineff S, Goldberg R, et al. Acute myocardial infarction as a complication of clonidine withdrawal. J Emerg Med 2003;25(4):399–402.
18. Geyskes GG, Boer P, Dorhout Mees EJ. Clonidine withdrawal. Mechanism and frequency of rebound hypertension. Br J Clin Pharmacol 1979;7(1):55–62.
19. Berge KH, Lanier WL. Myocardial infarction accompanying acute clonidine withdrawal in a patient without a history of ischemic coronary artery disease. Anesth Analg 1991;72(2):259–61.
20. Judge R, Parry MG, Quail D, et al. Discontinuation symptoms: comparison of brief interruption in fluoxetine and paroxetine treatment. Int Clin Psychopharmacol 2002;17(5):217–25.
21. Haddad PM. Antidepressant discontinuation syndromes. Drug Saf 2001;24(3): 183–97.
22. Jasinska-Stroschein M, Owczarek J, Wejman I, et al. Novel mechanistic and clinical implications concerning the safety of statin discontinuation. Pharmacol Rep 2011;63(4):867–79.
23. Endres M, Laufs U. Discontinuation of statin treatment in stroke patients. Stroke 2006;37(10):2640–3.

24. Jabbour SA. Steroids and the surgical patient. Med Clin North Am 2001;85(5): 1311–7.
25. Mirski MA, Varelas PN. Seizures and status epilepticus in the critically ill. Crit Care Clin 2008;24(1):115–47, ix.
26. Castilla-Guerra L, del Carmen Fernandez-Moreno M, Lopez-Chozas JM, et al. Electrolytes disturbances and seizures. Epilepsia 2006;47(12):1990–8.
27. Miller AD, Ball AM, Bookstaver PB, et al. Epileptogenic potential of carbapenem agents: mechanism of action, seizure rates, and clinical considerations. Pharmacotherapy 2011;31(4):408–23.
28. Wong VK, Wright HT Jr, Ross LA, et al. Imipenem/cilastatin treatment of bacterial meningitis in children. Pediatr Infect Dis J 1991;10(2):122–5.
29. Wallace KL. Antibiotic-induced convulsions. Crit Care Clin 1997;13(4):741–62.
30. Pisani F, Oteri G, Costa C, et al. Effects of psychotropic drugs on seizure threshold. Drug Saf 2002;25(2):91–110.
31. Kahn LH, Alderfer RJ, Graham DJ. Seizures reported with tramadol. JAMA 1997;278(20):1661.
32. Talaie H, Panahandeh R, Fayaznouri M, et al. Dose-independent occurrence of seizure with tramadol. J Med Toxicol 2009;5(2):63–7.
33. Latta KS, Ginsberg B, Barkin RL. Meperidine: a critical review. Am J Ther 2002; 9(1):53–68.
34. Thundiyil JG, Kearney TE, Olson KR. Evolving epidemiology of drug-induced seizures reported to a Poison Control Center System. J Med Toxicol 2007;3(1): 15–9.
35. De Sarro A, Ammendola D, Zappala M, et al. Relationship between structure and convulsant properties of some beta-lactam antibiotics following intracerebroventricular microinjection in rats. Antimicrob Agents Chemother 1995;39(1): 232–7.
36. Akahane K, Sekiguchi M, Une T, et al. Structure-epileptogenicity relationship of quinolones with special reference to their interaction with gamma-aminobutyric acid receptor sites. Antimicrob Agents Chemother 1989;33(10):1704–8.
37. Raichle ME, Kutt H, Louis S, et al. Neurotoxicity of intravenously administered penicillin G. Arch Neurol 1971;25(3):232–9.
38. Calandra GB, Ricci FM, Wang C, et al. The efficacy results and safety profile of imipenem/cilastatin from the clinical research trials. J Clin Pharmacol 1988; 28(2):120–7.
39. Montgomery SA. Antidepressants and seizures: emphasis on newer agents and clinical implications. Int J Clin Pract 2005;59(12):1435–40.
40. Gill KV, Voils SA, Chenault GA, et al. Perceived versus actual sedation practices in adult intensive care unit patients receiving mechanical ventilation. Ann Pharmacother 2012;46(10):1331–9.
41. Pandharipande PP, Pun BT, Herr DL, et al. Effect of sedation with dexmedetomidine vs lorazepam on acute brain dysfunction in mechanically ventilated patients: the MENDS randomized controlled trial. JAMA 2007;298(22):2644–53.
42. Riker RR, Shehabi Y, Bokesch PM, et al. Dexmedetomidine vs midazolam for sedation of critically ill patients: a randomized trial. JAMA 2009;301(5):489–99.
43. Barr J, Fraser GL, Puntillo K, et al. Clinical practice guidelines for the management of pain, agitation, and delirium in adult patients in the intensive care unit. Crit Care Med 2013;41(1):263–306.
44. Naber D, Sand P, Heigl B. Psychopathological and neuropsychological effects of 8-days' corticosteroid treatment. A prospective study. Psychoneuroendocrinology 1996;21(1):25–31.

45. Brown ES, Chandler PA. Mood and cognitive changes during systemic cortico-steroid therapy. Prim Care Companion J Clin Psychiatry 2001;3(1):17–21.

46. Fardet L, Petersen I, Nazareth I. Suicidal behavior and severe neuropsychiatric disorders following glucocorticoid therapy in primary care. Am J Psychiatry 2012;169(5):491–7.

47. Lewis DA, Smith RE. Steroid-induced psychiatric syndromes. A report of 14 cases and a review of the literature. J Affect Disord 1983;5(4):319–32.

48. Schreiber MP, Colantuoni E, Bienvenu OJ, et al. Corticosteroids and transition to delirium in patients with acute lung injury. Crit Care Med 2014;42(6):1480–6.

49. Acute adverse reactions to prednisone in relation to dosage. Clin Pharmacol Ther 1972;13(5):694–8.

50. Cantu TG, Korek JS. Central nervous system reactions to histamine-2 receptor blockers. Ann Intern Med 1991;114(12):1027–34.

51. Roberts DJ, Hall RI, Kramer AH, et al. Sedation for critically ill adults with severe traumatic brain injury: a systematic review of randomized controlled trials. Crit Care Med 2011;39(12):2743–51.

52. Albanese J, Viviand X, Potie F, et al. Sufentanil, fentanyl, and alfentanil in head trauma patients: a study on cerebral hemodynamics. Crit Care Med 1999;27(2):407–11.

53. Warner DS, Hindman BJ, Todd MM, et al. Intracranial pressure and hemody-namic effects of remifentanil versus alfentanil in patients undergoing supraten-torial craniotomy. Anesth Analg 1996;83(2):348–53.

54. Tipps LB, Coplin WM, Murry KR, et al. Safety and feasibility of continuous infu-sion of remifentanil in the neurosurgical intensive care unit. Neurosurgery 2000;46(3):596–601 [discussion: 601–2].

55. Girard F, Moumdjian R, Boudreault D, et al. The effect of sedation on intracranial pressure in patients with an intracranial space-occupying lesion: remifentanil versus propofol. Anesth Analg 2009;109(1):194–8.

56. Brown MM, Parr MJ, Manara AR. The effect of suxamethonium on intracranial pressure and cerebral perfusion pressure in patients with severe head injuries following blunt trauma. Eur J Anaesthesiol 1996;13(5):474–7.

57. Clancy M, Halford S, Walls R, et al. In patients with head injuries who undergo rapid sequence intubation using succinylcholine, does pretreatment with a competitive neuromuscular blocking agent improve outcome? A literature re-view. Emerg Med J 2001;18(5):373–5.

58. Stirt JA, Grosslight KR, Bedford RF, et al. "Defasciculation" with metocurine pre-vents succinylcholine-induced increases in intracranial pressure. Anesthesi-ology 1987;67(1):50–3.

59. Silber SH. Rapid sequence intubation in adults with elevated intracranial pres-sure: a survey of emergency medicine residency programs. Am J Emerg Med 1997;15(3):263–7.

60. Cottrell JE, Patel K, Turndorf H, et al. Intracranial pressure changes induced by sodium nitroprusside in patients with intracranial mass lesions. J Neurosurg 1978;48(3):329–31.

61. Griswold WR, Reznik V, Mendoza SA. Nitroprusside-induced intracranial hyper-tension. JAMA 1981;246(23):2679–80.

62. Anile C, Zanghi F, Bracali A, et al. Sodium nitroprusside and intracranial pres-sure. Acta Neurochir (Wien) 1981;58(3–4):203–11.

63. Suri MF, Vazquez G, Ezzeddine MA, et al. A multicenter comparison of out-comes associated with intravenous nitroprusside and nicardipine treatment among patients with intracerebral hemorrhage. Neurocrit Care 2009;11(1):50–5.

64. Lagerkranser M. Effects of nitroglycerin on intracranial pressure and cerebral blood flow. Acta Anaesthesiol Scand Suppl 1992;97:34–6.
65. Gagnon RL, Marsh ML, Smith RW, et al. Intracranial hypertension caused by nitroglycerin. Anesthesiology 1979;51(1):86–7.
66. Ohar JM, Fowler AA, Selhorst JB, et al. Intravenous nitroglycerin-induced intracranial hypertension. Crit Care Med 1985;13(10):867–8.
67. Skinhoj E, Overgaard J. Effect of dihydralazine on intracranial pressure in patients with severe brain damage. Acta Med Scand Suppl 1983;678:83–7.
68. Gaab MR, Czech T, Korn A. Intracranial effects of nicardipine. Br J Clin Pharmacol 1985;20(Suppl 1):67S–74S.
69. Nishiyama T, Yokoyama T, Matsukawa T, et al. Continuous nicardipine infusion to control blood pressure after evacuation of acute cerebral hemorrhage. Can J Anaesth 2000;47(12):1196–201.
70. Graffagnino C, Riker RR, Bergese S, et al. Assessment of cerebral perfusion pressure (CPP) and intracranial pressure (ICP) in patients with acute intracerebral hemorrhage (ICH) receiving aggressive blood pressure management with clevidipine: an analysis from the accelerate trial (a single-arm, open-label study of clevidipine). Neurocrit Care 2010;13:S93.
71. Olsen KS, Svendsen LB, Larsen FS, et al. Effect of labetalol on cerebral blood flow, oxygen metabolism and autoregulation in healthy humans. Br J Anaesth 1995;75(1):51–4.
72. Van Aken H, Puchstein C, Schweppe ML, et al. Effect of labetalol on intracranial pressure in dogs with and without intracranial hypertension. Acta Anaesthesiol Scand 1982;26(6):615–9.
73. Roush MK, Nelson KM. Understanding drug-induced febrile reactions. Am Pharm 1993;NS33(10):39–42.
74. Tabor PA. Drug-induced fever. Drug Intell Clin Pharm 1986;20(6):413–20.
75. Hanson MA. Drug fever. Remember to consider it in diagnosis. Postgrad Med 1991;89(5):167–70, 173.
76. Mackowiak PA, LeMaistre CF. Drug fever: a critical appraisal of conventional concepts. An analysis of 51 episodes in two Dallas hospitals and 97 episodes reported in the English literature. Ann Intern Med 1987;106(5):728–33.
77. Harris LF, Holdsambeck HK. Drug fever–surprisingly common and costly. Ala Med 1986;56(3):19–22.
78. Cacoub P, Musette P, Descamps V, et al. The DRESS syndrome: a literature review. Am J Med 2011;124(7):588–97.
79. Cluff LE, Johnson JE. Drug fever. Prog Allergy 1964;8:149–94.
80. Johnson DH, Cunha BA. Drug fever. Infect Dis Clin North Am 1996;10(1):85–91.

Brain Death and Management of a Potential Organ Donor in the Intensive Care Unit

Teddy S. Youn, MD, David M. Greer, MD, MA*

KEYWORDS

- Brain death • Intensive care unit • Organ donation • Ethics • Communication

KEY POINTS

- The concept of brain death developed with the advent of mechanical ventilation, and guidelines for determining brain death have been refined over time.
- The most current guidelines, the 2010 American Academy of Neurology practice parameters for brain death determination in adults, necessitate 3 clinical findings: irreversible coma from a known cause, brainstem areflexia, and apnea.
- Despite efforts to develop standardized guidelines, there is a large degree of practice variability, including the role of ancillary testing.
- Organ donation after brain death is a common source of transplant organs in Western countries. Early identification and notification of organ procurement organizations are essential. Management of potential organ donors must take into consideration specific pathophysiologic changes (eg, hemodynamics, hormonal production, and inflammation) for medical optimization.
- Philosophical, medicolegal, and ethical/religious debates about concerns regarding the relationship of brain death determination with organ donation, and whether or not brain death equates to death by any other definition, make communication with families key to assuaging any distrust of medical providers. The family meeting is a critical time to be compassionate and to skillfully educate the family as to what it means when their relative becomes brain dead.

INTRODUCTION

The concept of brain death has developed remarkably over the years (**Table 1**). As early as the 12th century, Rabbi Moses Maimonides, an intellectual figure of medieval

Conflicts of Interest: The authors have no relevant conflicts of interest to declare.
Disclosures: None.
Department of Neurology, Yale University School of Medicine, LLCI 912, 15 York Street, New Haven, CT 06520, USA
* Corresponding author.
E-mail address: david.greer@yale.edu

Crit Care Clin 30 (2014) 813–831
http://dx.doi.org/10.1016/j.ccc.2014.06.010   criticalcare.theclinics.com
0749-0704/14/$ – see front matter © 2014 Elsevier Inc. All rights reserved.

Table 1
Variation in the implementation of neurologic criteria to diagnose death in Australia, Canada, and the United Kingdom

	Australia	Canada	United Kingdom
Concept	Brain is defined as unresponsive coma, brainstem areflexia, absence of respiratory center function, in the clinical setting in which these findings are irreversible Brain death is determined by: clinical testing; or imaging that shows the absence of intracranial blood flow. However, no clinical or imaging tests can establish that every brain cell has died	Brain death is defined as the irreversible loss of the capacity for consciousness combined with the irreversible loss of all brainstem functions, including the capacity to breathe	When the brainstem has been damaged in such a way, and to such a degree, that its integrative functions (which include the neural control of cardiac and pulmonary function and consciousness) are irreversibly destroyed, the individual has died
Cause	Evidence of sufficient intracranial disease to cause whole brain death. Brain death cannot be determined when the condition causing coma and loss of all brainstem function has affected only the brainstem, and there is still blood flow to the supratentorial part of the brain	Established cause capable of causing neurologic death There must be definite clinical or neuroimaging evidence of an acute CNS event consistent with the irreversible loss of neurologic function	There should be no doubt that the patient's condition is caused by irreversible brain damage of known cause
Minimum observation period before clinical testing	4 h; in cases of acute anoxic ischemic brain injury, clinical testing for brain death should be delayed for 24 h after the cardiorespiratory arrest	Any time after exclusion of confounders In cases of acute anoxic ischemic brain injury, clinical evaluation should be delayed for 24 h after the cardiorespiratory arrest, or an ancillary test could be performed	Left to the clinician to be satisfied that the patient's condition is the result of irreversible brain damage of known cause

	Australia	Canada	United Kingdom
Medical personnel who can confirm death	Two medical practitioners. Qualifications and experience requirements vary between each state in Australia	Recommended minimum level of physician qualification is full and current licensure for independent medical practice in the relevant Canadian jurisdiction and possessing skill and knowledge in the management of patients with severe brain injury and in the neurologic determination of death	Two medical practitioners who have been registered for >5 y and are competent in the conduct and interpretation of brainstem testing. ≤1 of the doctors must be a consultant
Repetition of tests	Each medical practitioner must separately carry out a clinical examination, so that the doctors and the tests are seen to be truly independent. The tests may be performed consecutively but not simultaneously	Two clinical tests at no fixed interval, 1 apnea test if performed concurrently with both physicians present. If performed at different times, a full clinical examination including the apnea test must be performed, without any fixed examination interval, regardless of the primary cause	Testing should be performed completely and successfully on 2 occasions with both doctors present
Apnea of test	Apnea must persist in the presence of an adequate stimulus to spontaneous ventilation (ie, an arterial $Paco_2$ >60 mm Hg and an arterial pH <7.30). The period of observation to achieve an adequate threshold of stimulus of the respiratory center is variable	Thresholds at completion of the apnea test: $Paco_2$ ≥60 mm Hg and ≥20 mm Hg higher than the pre-apnea test level and pH ≤7.28, as determined by arterial blood gases	$Paco_2$ >45 mm Hg and pH <7.4 before disconnection from mechanical ventilation followed by 5 min of observed apnea, confirming that the $Paco_2$ has increased by more than 4 mm Hg
Role of confirmatory investigation	If clinical testing cannot be relied on because preconditions are not met, absence of intracranial blood flow is diagnostic	An ancillary test should be performed when it is impossible to complete the minimum clinical criteria	In instances in which a comprehensive neurologic examination is not possible, in which a primary metabolic or pharmacologic derangement cannot be ruled out, or in cases of high cervical cord injury
Recommended confirmatory investigation	Demonstration of absence of intracranial blood flow. Four-vessel angiography and radionuclide imaging are the preferred imaging techniques for assessing intracranial blood flow	Evidence of the global absence of intracerebral blood flow. EEG is no longer recommended	None specifically recommended

The United States is not listed here; there is no national standard.

Adapted from Gardiner D, Shemie S, Manara A, et al. International perspective on the diagnosis of death. Br J Anaesth 2012;108(51):i14–28; with permission.

Judaism, argued that the spasmodic jerking observed in decapitated humans did not represent evidence of life, because the movements clearly did not originate from the brain: an argument that may represent the beginnings of the concept of brain death.[1] In 1664, Thomas Willis in his text, *Cerebri Anatome*, was able to elucidate specific cerebral functions by autopsy of deceased patients, where he argued that the brain ruled over other parts of the body, and the nerves carried out the actions.[2] However, the concept of brain death remained theoretic before the 1950s, because patients who suffered a devastating brain injury proceeded quickly to respiratory and cardiac arrest.[3] The advent of positive pressure ventilation in 1952 by Bjorn Ibsen allowed for the continued support of comatose patients.[4] In 1959, Pierre Mollaret and Maurice Goulon, neurologists at Claude Bernard Hospital in Paris, published an article, "Le coma dépassé," which described "irretrievable coma" in artificially ventilated patients and laid the groundwork for the development of clinical criteria for brain death.[5] The description of this type of coma prompted the investigators and others to ask whether continued care in these cases was necessary or appropriate. From these seminal early works, it became clear that physicians were unsure whether patients with *coma dépassé* were alive or dead, and that a reevaluation of what it meant to be dead in this new technological era was required.[6]

BRAIN DEATH CRITERIA
Practice Before the American Academy of Neurology Guidelines

In 1968, a committee commissioned by Harvard Medical School involving physicians, a theologian, a lawyer, and a historian of science examined irreversible coma as a new criterion for death.[7] In their report, coma in an individual with no discernible central nervous system (CNS) activity was defined by 4 features: (1) unreceptivity and unresponsiveness; (2) absent movements or breathing; (3) absent reflexes; and (4) an isoelectric electroencephalogram (EEG).[8] Confounders such as hypothermia (<32.2°C [90°F]) or the presence of CNS depressants need to be corrected or excluded to diagnose brain death. These professionals recommended confirmation of these findings by a second examination at least 24 hours after the first examination. This was the first formal attempt to codify anatomic criteria for determining how someone may be brain dead even though the heart may continue to beat. It was later suggested that brain death should be a clinical diagnosis and not rely on electrodiagnostic testing.[9,10] In addition, testing for apnea, exclusion of metabolic derangements, and a shorter period until the second examination were included in the later Minnesota criteria. In 1977, an effort to standardize these criteria was initiated by the National Institutes of Health–sponsored multicenter US Collaborative Study of Cerebral Death.[11,12] This study recommended 2 separate examinations, the second at least 6 hours from the time of onset of coma and including apnea testing. The examinations needed to show cerebral unresponsiveness, dilated unreactive pupils, absent brainstem reflexes, apnea, and an isoelectric EEG.

The United Kingdom concurrently charged a multidisciplinary working group, the Joint Committee of the Royal Colleges of Physicians, to formulate criteria for brain death.[13] The UK criteria were the first to argue that "...permanent functional death of the brainstem constitutes brain death," a variation that remains controversial.[14] The history and implications of this difference is beyond the scope of this article but is well reviewed in the literature.[15]

In 1981, the President's Commission for the Study of Ethical Problems in Medicine and Biomedical and Behavioral Research published a report delineating guidelines on brain death determination that represented a distillation of the practice at that time. The chair of this commission, Morris Abram, wrote that "... in light of the ever increasing powers of biomedical science and practice, a statute is needed to provide a clear and socially acceptable basis for making determinations of death."[16] These guidelines became the gold standard for more than a decade in the United States, and became the medical rationale for the legal framework for the Uniform Determination of Death Act (UDDA).[17] It states: "An individual who has sustained either (1) irreversible cessation of circulatory and respiratory functions, or (2) irreversible cessation of all functions of the entire brain, including the brain stem, is dead. A determination of death must be made in accordance with accepted medical standards."

This law differs substantially from laws determining brain death in other countries that specify exactly which medical judgments and tests are written into legal statutes.[18] This law allows for variation in interpretation and practice in the determination of brain death in the United States. UDDA has been adopted in 45 states and recognized in the rest through judicial opinion.

The American Academy of Neurology Guidelines (1995 and the 2010 Update)

In light of the variability in criteria for determining brain death, the American Academy of Neurology (AAN) developed practice parameters with a standard protocol in 1995.[19] This methodical approach for the clinical diagnosis of death by neurologic criteria involves (1) documentation of loss of consciousness, (2) absence of motor response to pain stimuli, (3) absence of brainstem reflexes, and (4) apnea.[20] The prerequisites for proceeding with the clinical diagnosis consisted of clinical or neuroimaging evidence of an acute CNS catastrophe compatible with the clinical diagnosis of brain death, the exclusion of confounding medical conditions (electrolyte, acid-base, or endocrine derangements), absence of drug intoxication or poisoning, and a core temperature of at least 32°C. This publication[20] is the foundation for the current practice of declaring brain death in neurologically devastated patients.

In 2010, the AAN published an update focusing on several clinical questions, including the potential for misdiagnosis, defining adequate observation times, the implications of complex motor movements, and the potential use of new ancillary tests.[21] The 2010 guidelines updated the previous guidelines and provided a clear algorithmic approach to brain death determination by emphasizing 3 key elements: irreversible coma (from a known proximate cause), brainstem areflexia, and coma. This update[21] also noted that: (1) no recoveries after the diagnosis of brain death had been shown since the adoption of the AAN 1995 guidelines, if the guidelines were followed correctly; (2) the apnea test had been refined over time and is safe using standardized oxygenation methods; (3) confirmatory tests are less reliable and useful than has been suggested and should be used sparingly; and (4) adequate documentation may be facilitated with a checklist. **Box 1** summarizes the steps for the determination of brain death.

Practice Variability in Brain Death Determination

Despite these efforts, there remains significant variation in practice regarding determination of brain death. A review of brain death policies at some of the top institutions of neurology and neurosurgery within the United States[22] reported wide practice inconsistencies both anecdotally in provider experiences and systematically within institutional policies. Discrepancies were noted with regard to which prerequisites should be met, the lowest acceptable core temperature, the number of examiners required, core features of the neurologic examination, methods of performing the apnea test, and when ancillary tests are implemented. Although national and international variability is extensive, even within a single institution there can be wide variability over which clinical tests are documented.[23] This lack of standardization has led to confusion in medical providers and fostered mistrust in the lay public. Therefore, the onus should be not only to establish strict, conservative, and comprehensive guidelines but also to encourage rigorous and uniform adoption of such guidelines.

Box 1
Checklist for determination of brain death

A. Prerequisites (all must be checked)
- Coma, irreversible and cause known
- Neuroimaging explains coma
- CNS-depressant drug effect absent (if indicated toxicology screen; if barbiturates given, serum level <10 µg/mL)
- No evidence of residual paralytics (electrical stimulation if paralytics are used)
- Absence of severe acid-base, electrolyte, endocrine abnormality
- Normothermia or mild hypothermia (core temperature >36°C)
- Systolic blood pressure 100 mm Hg or greater
- No spontaneous respirations

B. Examination (all must be checked)
- Pupils nonreactive to bright light
- Corneal reflex absent
- Oculocephalic reflex absent (tested only if C-spine integrity is ensured)
- Oculovestibular reflex absent
- No facial movement to noxious stimuli at supraorbital nerve, temporomandibular joint
- Gag reflex absent
- Cough reflex absent to tracheal suctioning
- Absence of motor response to noxious stimuli in all 4 limbs (spinally mediated reflexes are permissible)

C. Apnea testing (all must be checked)
- Patient is hemodynamically stable (even with the use of vasopressors)
- Ventilator adjusted to provide normocarbia ($Paco_2$ 35–45 mm Hg)
- Patient preoxygenated with 100% Fio_2 for greater than 10 minutes to Pao_2 greater than 200 mm Hg
- Patient well oxygenated with a positive end-expiratory pressure of 5 cm of water
- Provide oxygen via a suction catheter to the level of the carina at 6 L/min or attach T-piece with continuous positive airway pressure at 10 cm H_2O
- Disconnect ventilator
- Spontaneous respirations absent
- Arterial blood gas drawn at 8 to 10 minutes, patient reconnected to ventilator
- $Paco_2$ 60 mm Hg or greater, or 20 mm Hg increase from normal baseline value
  or
- Apnea test aborted

D. Ancillary testing (only 1 needs to be performed; to be ordered only if clinical examination cannot be fully performed because of patient factors, or if apnea testing inconclusive, contraindicated, or aborted)

- Cerebral angiogram

- Hexamethylpropyleneamine oxime single-photon emission computed tomography

- EEG

- Transcranial Doppler

Adapted from Wijdicks EF, Varelas PN, Gronseth GS, et al. American Academy of Neurology. Evidence-based guideline update: determining brain death in adults: report of the Quality Standards Subcommittee of the American Academy of Neurology. Neurology 2010;74:1917; with permission.

Common Pitfalls in Determination

No published peer-reviewed cases of clinical mimics of brain death have detailed a full neurologic brain death examination according to the AAN practice guidelines. In most of the frequently cited cases of brain death mimics, high cervical cord injury,[24] fulminant Guillain-Barré syndrome,[25,26] organophosphate intoxication,[27] baclofen overdose,[28] barbiturate overdose,[29] lidocaine toxicity,[30] and delayed vecuronium clearance[31] were the diagnoses that were the most common for a clinical diagnosis mimicking brain death. However, in reviewing those cases, all had at least 1 violation of the AAN practice guidelines on brain death determination. Thus, when used correctly and supported by ancillary testing when necessary, the AAN practice guidelines for brain death determination correctly diagnose brain death with absolute certainty.

Several clinical signs should warn against possible premature assessment for brain death, including normal neuroimaging, normotension without vasopressor support, absence of diabetes insipidus, marked heart rate variations, fever, marked metabolic acidosis, hypothermia lower than 32°C, marked miosis (opiate or organophosphate toxicity), myoclonus (lithium or selective serotonin reuptake inhibitor [SSRI] toxicity), rigidity (SSRI or haloperidol toxicity), profuse sweating (organophosphates), abnormal laboratory values, or positive toxicology (either urine or serum).[3]

The 2 most common confounders are drug intoxication and hypothermia. Excluding the effect of sedative medications usually requires the calculation of clearance of at least 5 times the known half-life of the drug when hepatic and renal function are normal and there is no influence of hypothermia. After ingestion or administration of an unknown, nonquantifiable substance, one should wait at least 48 hours before brain death examination (**Table 2**).

Hypothermia can lead to a progressive loss of neurologic function, including brainstem reflexes.[32] Pupillary dilatation and sluggish pupillary responses occur at core temperatures between 28°C and 32°C, and other brainstem reflexes disappear lower than 28°C.[33] Coingestion of drugs such as opioids, benzodiazepines, phenothiazines, tricyclic antidepressants, and lithium may all contribute to hypothermia and should be considered if a patient is unexpectedly hypothermic.[3] Successful resuscitation after slow rewarming has recently been reported with good cognitive outcome in a patient who had a temperature of 13.7°C.[34] For these reasons, strict adherence to the AAN guidelines is necessary to ensure proper evaluation of patients for brain death.

A common misconception in the diagnosis of brain death is that patients who are dead by neurologic criteria (ie, brain dead) should have no movement. Movements in brain death are common and have a wide range of phenomenology.[35,36] Although

Table 2
Half-life (in hours) of some CNS-depressant drugs

Amitriptyline	24
Atracurium	0.5
Clonazepam	20
Codeine	3
Diazepam	40
Fentanyl	6
Ketamine	2.5
Lorazepam	15
Midazolam	6
Morphine	3
Pancuronium	2
Phenobarbital	100
Primidone	20
Rocuronium	1
Thiopental	20
Vecuronium	2

Data from Wijdicks EF. Brain death. Oxford (United Kingdom): Oxford University Press; 2011.

evidence points to hypoxic injury of spinal neurons for these movements, the pathophysiology for many cases is speculative. Most reported reflexes and automatisms associated with brain death can be triggered by stimulation, such as neck flexion, noxious stimulus, and apnea testing. They are also time dependent, emerging or resolving at specific time points after the onset of brain death. Recognizing spinally mediated movements and differentiating them from purposeful movements requires expertise, and sometimes, ancillary testing may be required when there is still doubt whether a movement might be cerebrally mediated. Failure to recognize spinally mediated movements may lead to confusion about the diagnosis by providers, distress to family members who witness these movements, and delay or even failure to fulfill a patient/family's wishes for organ donation.

Ancillary Testing

Apnea testing is the definitive test for brain death in a patient who meets the other established clinical criteria. Risks of complications from apnea testing are varied, mostly involving complications of hypoxemia, hypotension, or cardiac arrhythmias.[37–39] The need for early termination of apnea testing is usually caused by failure to preoxygenate, lack of oxygen administration during testing, high intratracheal flow of oxygen (>10 L/min), which washes out carbon dioxide and leads to failure to achieve an increased $Paco_2$, high alveolar-arterial gradient (>300), mild acidosis (arterial pH <7.30), chest tubes for pneumothorax, polytrauma, and younger age.[3] An ancillary test may be necessary when apnea testing cannot be performed because of uncorrectable toxic levels of confounding medications, hemodynamic or pulmonary instability, or conditions resulting in chronic retention of carbon dioxide, as in sleep apnea or severe pulmonary disease.[39] An ancillary test is essential in patients in whom brainstem reflexes cannot be adequately tested, as is the case with severe facial trauma or preexisting bilateral pupillary abnormalities. However, in the United States, when the clinical criteria for brain death determination are satisfied in entirety, ancillary testing is not required in adults. This situation is not always true internationally. However, ancillary testing should never supersede the clinical examination in brain death determination.

Validated ancillary tests are divided into those that test the electrical function of the brain and those that test cerebral blood flow (**Box 2**). These tests include digital subtraction cerebral angiography, transcranial Doppler ultrasonography, EEG, and nuclear cerebral blood flow scanning. False-positive and false-negative tests can occur.[40] **Box 2** represents the AAN's summary of allowed ancillary tests. Methods such as magnetic resonance angiography, computed tomography angiography, somatosensory evoked potentials, and bispectral index are not accepted because of insufficient evidence to support their use in brain death determination.

Documentation

Once brain death is determined in a patient, the time of brain death is documented in the medical record.[21] The recorded time of death is the official laboratory time that the arterial P_{CO_2} reached the target value during apnea testing. In patients who undergo ancillary testing as their means of determination, the time of death is when the ancillary test is officially interpreted. Although documentation of brain death testing should uniformly state requisite clinical conditions, clinical examination findings, and apnea or ancillary testing results, wide variability has been found in the literature. In 2002, a retrospective review of brain death declarations at a single, major medical center[23] was analyzed; testing of different cranial nerves was variably documented regarding pupillary light (86%), gag (78%), and corneal (57%) reflexes. More recently in 2011, researchers at the University of Chicago[41] found that of 68 heterogeneous hospitals in the Midwest, only 45.1% of 226 brain-dead organ donors had complete documentation of brainstem areflexia and absent motor responses. Apnea testing was completed in 73.5%. Of the 60 without completed apnea testing, 93.3% had ancillary testing consistent with brain death. Overall, only 44.7% strictly adhered to AAN guidelines. Uniformity in documentation is essential to develop trustworthiness as providers to the lay public, and the efficiency of the courts depends on an accurate diagnosis of brain death and the time of death.[42]

MANAGEMENT OF POTENTIAL ORGAN DONOR

Patients in the intensive care unit (ICU) declared dead by neurologic criteria (or by circulatory criteria) are potential organ donors. Because of the shortage of available organs for donation, optimizing appropriate management of potential donors is of great importance.[43–47] One donor has the potential to affect the lives of 7 or more people.

Identification of Potential Organ Donors and Organ Procurement Organizations

The Uniform Anatomic Gift Act of 1968,[48] which grants individuals older than 18 years the power to donate their own organ and tissue, was accepted by all states in 1972 and led to the National Organ Transplant Act of 1984,[49] which developed a national organ transplant system, known as the Organ Procurement and Transplantation Network (OPTN).[50] The Health Care Financing Administration in 1986 awarded the private, nonprofit organization, United Network for Organ Sharing (UNOS), a contract to operate OPTN. UNOS now administers more than 58 federally regulated organ procurement organizations (OPOs). OPOs are responsible as the liaisons between local hospitals and UNOS and are responsible for procuring, preserving, and allocating all organs and tissues. Procurement of organs and tissue after the clinical diagnosis of brain death is granted by families in more than 70% of cases when it is requested.[3]

Box 2
Methods of ancillary testing for the determination of brain death

A. Cerebral angiography

- The contrast medium should be injected in the aortic arch under high pressure and reach both anterior and posterior circulations.
- No intracerebral filling should be detected at the level of entry of the carotid or vertebral artery to the skull.
- The external carotid circulation should be patent.
- The filling of the superior longitudinal sinus may be delayed.

B. EEG

- A minimum of 8 scalp electrodes should be used.
- Interelectrode impedance should be between 100 and 10,000 Ohms.
- The integrity of the entire recording system should be tested.
- The distance between electrodes should be at least 10 cm.
- The sensitivity should be increased to at least 2 mV for 30 minutes, with inclusion of appropriate calibrations.
- The high-frequency filter setting should not be set lower than 30 Hz, and the low-frequency setting should not be higher than 1 Hz.
- EEG should show a lack of reactivity to intense somatosensory or audiovisual stimuli.

C. Transcranial Doppler ultrasonography

- Transcranial Doppler ultrasonography is useful only if a reliable signal is found. The abnormalities should include either reverberating flow or small systolic peaks in early systole. A finding of a complete absence of flow may not be reliable because of inadequate transtemporal windows for insonation. There should be bilateral insonation and anterior and posterior insonation. The probe should be placed at the temporal bone above the zygomatic arch and the vertebrobasilar arteries, through the suboccipital transcranial window. Two evaluations, at least 30 minutes apart, must be performed.
- Insonation through the orbital window can be considered to obtain a reliable signal. Transcranial Doppler ultrasonography may be less reliable in patients with a previous craniotomy.

D. Cerebral scintigraphy (technetium Tc99m exametazime [hexamethylpropyleneamine oxime])

- The isotope should be injected within 30 minutes after its reconstitution.
- Anterior and both lateral planar image counts (500,000) of the head should be obtained at several time points: immediately, between 30 and 60 minutes later, and at 2 hours.
- A correct intravenous injection may be confirmed with additional images of the liver showing uptake (optional).
- No radionuclide localization in the middle cerebral artery, anterior cerebral artery, or basilar artery territories of the cerebral hemispheres (hollow skull phenomenon).
- No tracer in superior sagittal sinus (minimal tracer can come from the scalp).

Adapted from Wijdicks EF, Varelas PN, Gronseth GS, et al. American Academy of Neurology. Evidence-based guideline update: determining brain death in adults: report of the Quality Standards Subcommittee of the American Academy of Neurology. Neurology 2010;74:1917; with permission.

The first step in moving care for brain-dead patients to possible organ donation is recognizing viable candidates early.[3] UNOS and other international organ procurement and transplantation networks have defined criteria for possible candidates under the following terms: (1) standard criteria donor: donors younger than 50 years who suffered brain death, and (2) expanded criteria donor: donors aged 60 years or older, or 50 to 59 years plus having 2 of the 3 following criteria: stroke or cardiac disease as the cause of death, hypertension, or a terminal serum creatinine level of greater than 1.5 mg/dL.[3,51,52] When a potential donor is identified, the local organ network should be notified immediately. These agencies become involved with a patient's family only after the treating staff make a clinical determination regarding prognosis, and all medical decisions must be totally independent from the patient's status regarding organ donation. After contact by the medical staff, the local OPO coordinator then determines medical suitability for possible organ donation.

Physicians involved in the medical care of the patients are not expected to screen patients for organ donation, and particular care must be taken to have no real or perceived conflicts of interest. Physicians are expected to inform the OPO representative whether a patient progresses to brain death or not. If the patient does not progress to brain death, but the decision is to withdraw supportive care because of irreversible brain damage, the OPO representative can obtain consent for organ donation from a surrogate before planned withdrawal from life-sustaining therapies. Organ procurement occurs after circulatory determination of death (DCDD); this is also known as nonheartbeating organ donation.[53]

The OPO representative, who is a trained requestor, should be the only one to have a specific discussion regarding possible consent for organ donation. Individuals involved in the transplantation process should never be involved in these discussions. General contraindications to organ donation are listed in **Box 3**.

Preparation for Organ Procurement

After consent for donation has been obtained, a detailed medical and social history and serologic and radiographic studies must be obtained to evaluate the viability of the potential organ donor; **Box 4** provides more details. In addition, a blood sample must be obtained for serologic testing, which must be completed before organ transplantation. Tissue typing and HLA identification are less critical but are necessary for allocation of donation of kidney and pancreas.

Pathophysiologic Changes After Brain Death and Medical Management

UNOS created a Critical Pathway for the Organ Donor in 1999, which recommended defined physiologic goals and a consistent and active approach to donor management, including treatments and monitoring.[54] The typical pathophysiologic consequences of brain death include dysfunction of the cardiovascular (hypotension, arrhythmias), pulmonary (pulmonary edema, ventilator-induced lung injury), endocrine (diabetes insipidus, hypoglycemia), thermoregulation (hypothermia), renal (acute kidney injury), hematologic (disseminated intravascular coagulation), and inflammatory (systemic inflammatory response) systems.[17] In addition, the systemic inflammatory response is more prominent than previously believed and may lead to poorer graft survival after transplantation.[55]

What follows is a set of recommendations that are typically used in optimizing medical management, including recommendations for hemodynamic medications (ie, inotropes, vasopressors), ventilator management, hormone replacement therapy (HRT), and thermoregulation support.

Box 3
Contraindications to organ donation

Infections

Bacterial

- Tuberculosis; gangrenous bowel, bowel perforation, intra-abdominal sepsis, multisystem organ failure caused by overwhelming sepsis

Viral

- Human immunodeficiency virus, rabies, varicella zoster virus, Epstein-Barr virus, West Nile virus, herpes simplex virus, and so forth
- Note: hepatitis B/hepatitis C virus organs and cytomegalovirus (+) organs can be transplanted into recipients, pending certain qualifications

Fungal

- *Cryptococcus, Aspergillus,* Histoplasmosis, *Coccidioides,* Candidemia

Parasitic

- Leishmaniasis, trypanosome, *Strongyloides,* malaria

Prion

- Creutzfeldt-Jakob disease and variants

General conditions

- Aplastic anemia
- Agranulocytosis
- Extreme immaturity (<500 g, or a gestational age of <32 weeks)
- Current malignancy except nonmelanoma skin cancers, primary CNS tumors without evident metastatic disease, and remote prostate cancer
- Previous malignancy with current evidence metastatic disease
- Previous melanoma
- Hematologic malignancies (eg, leukemia, lymphoma, multiple myeloma)

Data from Wijdicks EF. Brain Death. Oxford (United Kingdom): Oxford University Press; 2011. p. 108, with permission; and Frontera JA, Kalb T. How I manage the adult potential organ donor: donation after neurological death (Part 1). Neurocrit Care 2010;12:104.

Temperature Management

One of the consequences of brain death is that there is deprivation of arterial perfusion to the hypothalamus, leading to a disconnection of the hypothalamic-pituitary axis and loss of temperature regulation.[56] Current practice includes active warming to maintain a donor's temperature greater than 35°C before and during organ procurement.[57] It has been hypothesized that active rapid cooling of organs before circulatory arrest might improve organ viability in DCDD cases.[58]

Cardiovascular/Hemodynamics Management

Hemodynamic instability following brain death can usually be attributed to 3 main causes. First, a sympathetic surge preceding medullary damage in brain death leads to a catecholamine surge, resulting in hypertension, left ventricular dysfunction, cardiac stunning, neurogenic pulmonary edema, and arrhythmias.[59] Second, spinal cord infarction that follows herniation results in loss of sympathetic tone, resulting in

> **Box 4**
> **Pre–organ procurement checklist**
>
> Heart:
>
> - 12-lead electrocardiogram
> - Echocardiogram (transesophageal route preferred)
> - Coronary angiography
> - Swan-Ganz readings (optional)
> - Cardiology consultation
>
> Lungs:
>
> - Chest radiograph
> - Arterial blood gas
> - PEEP
> - Bronchoscopy
> - Oxygen challenge test
> - Pulmonary consultation
>
> Serologic tests:
>
> - Human immunodeficiency virus; hepatitis B/hepatitis C virus; cytomegalovirus; rapid plasma regain–*Treponema pallidum* agglutination testing
>
> Laboratory tests:
>
> - General (electrolytes, blood urea nitrogen, creatinine, glucose, complete blood count, calcium, magnesium, phosphorus)
> - Blood cultures
> - Liver tests (aspartate transaminase, alanine transaminase, bilirubin, γ-glutamyl transpeptidase, alkaline phosphatase, lactate dehydrogenase, coagulation tests)
> - Kidney (urinalysis, urine culture)
> - Heart (creatine phosphokinase, troponin)
> - Pancreas (amylase, lipase)
> - Lungs (sputum, Gram stain)
>
> *Data from* Wijdicks EF. Brain death. Oxford (United Kingdom): Oxford University Press; 2011. p. 109.

further hypotension. Third, pituitary dysfunction is common, because tissue shifts often damage the gland and can lead to a panhypopituitary state (see later discussion). Ensuing diabetes insipidus also leads to further hypotension as a result of hypovolemia. Management with a combination of fluid replacement, desmopressin, inotropes, or vasopressors is commonly used. Given the high association of concomitant diabetes insipidus in these patients, vasopressin is often the first-line vasopressor in potential donors. Regardless of the exact treatment plan, a mean arterial pressure greater than 60 mm Hg and urine output greater than 0.5 mL/kg/h should be maintained. Avoiding excessive fluid loading in donor management has consistently been shown to increase the numbers of transplantable lungs.[60] Studies are under way to determine if a protocolized fluid management of brain-dead donors, directed by pulse-pressure variation, can increase the viability of lungs and other organs.[61]

Myocardial dysfunction is common after brain death, and an early transthoracic echocardiogram should be performed to assess cardiac function. Patients with an ejection fraction less than 45% likely require inotropic support; norepinephrine is often the first agent of choice, although phenylephrine can also be used.[45] Stunned myocardium is not an uncommon feature after brain death; therefore, repeat echocardiography is frequently encouraged. In patients who are potential cardiac donors, coronary angiography may be required before donation, and if needed, it should be performed quickly to avoid delays in procurement, which have been shown to lower the yield of cardiac allografts.[62]

Pulmonary/Ventilator Management

Lungs may become damaged because of trauma, aspiration pneumonitis, and fat emboli.[63] True neurogenic pulmonary edema after the diagnosis of brain death is uncommon, can easily be managed with slightly higher levels of positive end-expiratory pressure (PEEP), and is usually fully reversible.[3] If a patient is a lung donor candidate, bronchoscopy should be performed to rule out any potential lesions or injury.

Lung damage from ventilator-induced lung injury in ICU patients is common.[64] Previously, high tidal volumes and low PEEP were commonly used for lung recruitment. Recent literature[65] has suggested that lung injury from brain-dead organ donors is similar to the injury seen in acute lung injury and acute respiratory distress syndrome. Lung protective ventilation strategies are the method of choice with potential lung organ donors, with tidal volumes of 6 to 8 mL/kg, a PEEP of 5 cm H_2O, and maneuvers to prevent derecruitment.[66]

Hormonal/Inflammatory Management

Multiple endocrine dysfunctions may occur after death by neurologic criteria as failure of the hypothalamus-pituitary axis occurs in the setting of severe hypoperfusion after brainstem herniation and intracranial hypertension. The posterior portion of the pituitary lobe is normally perfused through the inferior hypophyseal arteries from the cavernous section of the internal carotid artery. This extradural source of blood supply to the pituitary may explain why in some cases normal hormonal production may exist.[3] Diabetes insipidus is the most common hormonal abnormality after brain death and is defined as urine output in excess of 250 mL/h for greater than 2 hours and a urine specific gravity less than 1.005. Diabetes insipidus occurs in 46% to 87% of cases of brain death.[59] If a donor is at high risk of developing hypovolemia and cardiovascular collapse, a continuous infusion of vasopressin is used at doses between 0.5 and 1.0 milliunits/kg/h, depending on the degree of hypotension. If the patient is normotensive or hypertensive, desmopressin can be given instead, because it affects only the V2 receptors found in the renal collecting tubules.

For patients who also show signs of panhypopituitarism, treating for hypothyroidism, and adrenal insufficiency may also be warranted. The UNOS Critical Pathway for the Organ Donor suggests a protocol of HRT of levothyroxine, insulin, methylprednisolone, and possibly vasopressin when indicated, because HRT has been found to improve cardiac graft outcomes.[67] Hormone replacement medications used to treat brain-dead organ donors are summarized in **Table 3**. The remaining possible organs to be donated, including pancreas, liver, and kidneys, are optimized by stable hemodynamics, with a plan to procure the organs as soon as possible and minimize the risk of inflammation.

THE FAMILY MEETING

The family meeting is an important time to understand the patient's wishes, afford an opportunity to comfort the family, address their needs, and set the tone to deliver

Table 3
Hormone replacement pharmacologic agents

Medications	Dose (Intravenous)	Notes
Methylprednisolone	20–30 mg/kg	May need to be dosed every 8–12 h
Levothyroxine	0.8–1.4 μg/kg/h	May be bolused 1–5 μg/kg Can contribute large amounts of fluid at high doses
Triiodothyronine	0.05–0.2 μg/kg/h	
Regular insulin	0.05–0.1 units/kg/h	Need to monitor glucose Can use D50% if normoglycemic
Desmopressin (DDAVP)	2–4 μg	May be given as frequently as every hour Titrate for UOP 3–4 mL/h
Vasopressin	0.5–1 milliunits/kg/h	Titrate for mean arterial pressure >70 Titrate for UOP 3–4 mL/h

Abbreviation: UOP, urine output.
From Demetriades D, Lam L. Assessment, monitoring, and management of brain-dead potential organ donors in the USA. In: Novitzky D, Cooper DK, eds. The brain-dead organ donor: pathophysiology and management. New York: Springer Science+Business Media; 2013; with permission.

bad news in a compassionate manner, a hallmark of high-quality ICU care.[68] It is important to establish a relationship with the family before the discussion of brain death, preferably before brain death testing, so that the family can understand the treatment plan and steps that will be taken in the care of their loved one. Once a patient has been determined to be brain dead, a discussion with the family takes place that centers on letting the family know that their loved one has died, and the body and organs are being supported by artificial means. Clergy, social work, nursing, medical providers, and other active team members ideally should be present. The senior provider should inform the family in clear, nontechnical language that the patient is dead, and the time of death should be given. Despite preparatory conversations, families sometimes take this devastating news as unexpected, and the response is commonly an outpouring of grief. Adequate time should be allowed for family members to grieve and compose themselves, and it may be prudent to offer a recapitulation of the clinical course to answer any questions the family may have on the determination of brain death. Brain death is often a confusing concept to families, and explanations may need to be repeated multiple times. For example, in a survey in 1997 with the immediate next of kin of 164 medically suitable organ donor candidates 4 to 6 months after the patient's death, 52% of nondonor respondents stated that people who are brain dead can recover.[69] This study clearly points out the dangers of incomplete understanding by families. It is of utmost importance to be able to explain to families as clearly as possible what has happened to their loved one, and that they are medically and legally dead.

A recent randomized controlled trial even suggested that family members may benefit from witnessing the evaluation of brain death.[70] Sixty-six percent of those in the intervention group (eg, family present during brain death evaluation) achieved perfect postintervention understanding scores from a questionnaire about understanding of brain death, with no apparent impact on psychological well-being, compared with 20% of patients who were not exposed to the evaluation of brain death ($P = .02\%$). When families are assured by providers that their loved one is not abandoned during end-of-life care, that they do not suffer, and that the clinician supports the family's decision, family satisfaction increases.[71] Physicians and families may require more than 1 formal meeting to explain the process of brain death, which ensures goodwill between families and caregivers, and possibly improves decisions made toward organ donation after death by neurologic criteria.

SUMMARY

With technological advances such as positive pressure ventilation and organ transplantation, modern medicine has caused a reevaluation of our basic presuppositions about the biological phenomenon of death, for which society has constructed pragmatic, medical, moral, and legal policies.[72] Despite periodic controversy, a vast majority consensus exists on what constitutes brain death and which criteria are necessary in its determination. A similar consensus exists on the dead donor rule, which allows for physicians to manage the donor who fulfills criteria for death by brain death without any moral ambivalence. Future aims in the fields of intensive and neurocritical care medicine must include reducing practice variability in the operational guidelines for determination of brain death, as well as improving communication with families about the process of determining brain death, so that trust in the doctor-patient relationship can be fully ensured. A uniform international guideline seems elusive.

For those patients who fulfill brain death criteria and are potential organ donors, proactive management of the potential organ donor, including early notification of the local organ donor network, HRT, lung protective ventilation with aggressive pulmonary care, and intensive cardiac monitoring, may ensure optimal preservation and procurement of organs in a manner truly worthy of their gift.

REFERENCES

1. Bernat JL. Brain death. In: Ethical Issues in Neurology. Boston: Butterworth Heinemann; 2002. p. 253–386.
2. O'Connor JP. Thomas Willis and the background to Cerebri Anatome. J R Soc Med 2003;96:4.
3. Wijdicks EF. Brain death. Oxford (United Kingdom): Oxford University Press; 2011.
4. Laureys S. Death, unconsciousness and the brain. Nat Rev Neurosci 2005;6: 899–909.
5. Mollaret P, Goulon M. Le coma dépassé (memoire preliminaire). Rev Neurol 1959;101:3–15.
6. Bernat JL. The concept and practice of brain death. In: Progress in Brain Research, Vol 150, The Boundaries of Consciousness: Neurobiology and Neuropathology. Amsterdam: Elsevier; 2005.
7. Ad Hoc Committee. A definition of irreversible coma. Report of the Ad Hoc Committee of the Harvard Medical School to Examine the definition of brain death. JAMA 1968;205:337–40.
8. Hwang DY, Gilmore EJ, Greer DM. Assessment of brain death in the neurocritical care unit. Neurosurg Clin N Am 2013;24:469–82.
9. Adams RD, Jequier M. The brain death syndrome: hypoxemic panencephalopathy. Schweiz Med Wochenschr 1969;99:65–73.
10. Mohandas A, Chou SN. Brain death–a clinical and pathologic study. J Neurosurg 1971;35:211–8.
11. National Institute of Neurological and Communicative Disorders and Stroke (NINCDS). An appraisal of the criteria of cerebral death, a summary statement of a collaborative study. JAMA 1977;237:982–6.

12. National Institute of Neurological and Communicative Disorders and Stroke Monograph No: 24. The NINCDS Collaborative Study of Brain Death: NIH; 1980. JAMA 1977;237:982–6 [summary; reprint].
13. Conference of Medical Royal Colleges and Faculties of the United Kingdom. Diagnosis of brain death. BMJ 1976;2:1187–8.
14. Working group convened by the Royal College of Physicians. Criteria for the diagnosis of brain stem death: review by a working group convened by the Royal College of Physicians and endorsed by the Conference of Medical Royal Colleges and their Faculties in the United Kingdom. J R Coll Physicians Lond 1995;29:381–2.
15. Wijdicks EF. The transatlantic divide over brain death determination and the debate. Brain 2012;135:1321–31.
16. President's Commission for the Study of Ethical Problems in Medicine and Biomedical and Behavioral Research. Defining death: a report on the medical, legal, and ethical issues in the determination of death. Washington, DC: Government Printing Office; 1981.
17. Uniform Determination of Death Act. In: 12 uniform laws annotated 589 (West 1993 and West supp (1997)). United States: National Conference of Commissioners on Uniform State Laws. 1980.
18. Wijdicks EF. Brain death worldwide: accepted fact but no global consensus in diagnostic criteria. Neurology 2002;58:20–5.
19. The Quality Standards Subcommittee of the American Academy of Neurology. Practice parameters for determining brain death in adults (summary statement). Neurology 1995;45:1012–4.
20. Wijdicks EF. Determining brain death in adults. Neurology 1995;45:1003–11.
21. Wijdicks EF, Varelas PN, Gronseth GS, et al. Evidence-based guideline update: determining brain death in adults: report of the Quality Standards Subcommittee of the American Academy of Neurology. Neurology 2010;74:1911–8.
22. Greer DM, Varelas PN, Haque S, et al. Variability of brain death determination guidelines in leading US neurologic institutions. Neurology 2008;70:284–9.
23. Wang MY, Wallace P, Gruen JP. Brain death documentation: analysis and issues. Neurosurgery 2002;51:731–6.
24. Waters C, French G, Burt M. Difficulty in brainstem death testing in the presence of high spinal cord injury. Br J Anaesth 2004;92:760–4.
25. Rivas S, Douds G, Ostdahl R, et al. Fulminant Guillain-Barré syndrome after closed head injury: a potentially reversible cause of an ominous examination. Case report. J Neurosurg 2008;108:595–600.
26. Stojkovic T, Verdin M, Hurtevent J, et al. Guillain-Barré syndrome resembling brainstem death in a patient with brain injury. J Neurol 2001;248:430–2.
27. Peter J, Prabhakar A, Pichamuthu K. In-laws, insecticide–and a mimic of brain death. Lancet 2008;371:622.
28. Ostermann M, Young B, Sibbald W, et al. Coma mimicking brain death following baclofen overdose. Intensive Care Med 2000;26:1144–6.
29. Kirshbaum R, Carollo V. Reversible iso-electric EEG in barbiturate coma. JAMA 1970;212:1215.
30. Richard I, LaPointe M, Wax P, et al. Non-barbiturate, drug-induced reversible loss of brainstem reflexes. Neurology 1998;51:639–40.
31. Kainuma M, Miyake T, Kanno T. Extremely prolonged vecuronium clearance in a brain death case. Anesthesiology 2001;95:1023–4.
32. Fischbeck K, Simon R. Neurological manifestations of accidental hypothermia. Ann Neurol 1981;10:384–7.

33. Boyd J, Brugger H, Shuster M. Prognostic factors in avalanche resuscitation: a systematic review. Resuscitation 2010;10:384–7.
34. Gilbert M, Busund R, Skagseth A, et al. Resuscitation from accidental hypothermia of 13.7 degrees C with circulatory arrest. Lancet 2000;355:375–6.
35. Jain S, DeGeorgia M. Brain death-associated reflexes and automatisms. Neurocrit Care 2005;3:122–6.
36. Ropper AH. Unusual spontaneous movements in brain-dead patients. Neurology 1984;34:1089–92.
37. Goudreau JL, Wijdicks EF, Emery SF. Complications during apnea testing in the determination of brain death: predisposing factors. Neurology 2000;55:1045–8.
38. Jeret JS, Benjamin JL. Risk of hypotension during apnea testing. Arch Neurol 1994;51:595–9.
39. Wijdicks EF, Rabinstein AA, Manno EM, et al. Pronouncing brain death: contemporary practice and safety of the apnea test. Neurology 2008;71:1240–4.
40. Wijdicks EF. The case against confirmatory tests for determining brain death in adults. Neurology 2010;75:77–83.
41. Shappell CN, Frank JI, Husari K, et al. Practice variability in brain death determination: a call to action. Neurology 2013;81:2009–14.
42. Burkle CM, Schipper AM, Wijdicks EF. Brain death and the courts. Neurology 2011;76:837–41.
43. Wood KE, Becker BN, McCartney JG, et al. Care of the potential organ donor. N Engl J Med 2004;351:273–9.
44. Dare AJ, Bartlett AS, Fraser JF. Critical care of the potential organ donor. Curr Neurol Neurosci Rep 2012;2012(12):456–65.
45. Frontera JA, Kalb T. How I manage the adult potential organ donor: donation after neurological death (part 1). Neurocrit Care 2010;12:103–10.
46. Rech TH, Moraes RB, Crispim D, et al. Management of the brain-dead organ donor: a systematic review and meta-analysis. Transplantation 2013;95:966–74.
47. McKeown DW, Bonser R, Kellum J. Management of the heartbeating brain-dead organ donor. Br J Anaesth 2012;108:i96–107.
48. National Conference of Commissioners on Uniform State Laws. Uniform Anatomical Gift Act. 1968. p. 1–18.
49. National Organ Transplant Act. In: Public Law 98-507. United States of America. 1984. p. 2339–47.
50. Organ Procurement and Transplantation Network. Health Resources and Services Administration, HHS. Final rule. Fed Regist 1999;64:56650–61.
51. Truog RD, Miller FG, Halpern SD. The dead-donor rule and the future of organ donation. N Engl J Med 2013;369:1287–9.
52. Metzger RA, Delmonico FL, Feng S, et al. Expanded criteria donors for kidney transplantation. Am J Transplant 2003;3:114–25.
53. Bernat JL, D'Alessandro AM, Port FK, et al. Report of a National Conference on Donation after cardiac death. Am J Transplant 2006;6:281–91.
54. UNOS. Critical pathway for the organ donor. Available at: http://organdonor.gov/images/pdfs/acotapp3.pdf. Accessed April 15, 2014.
55. Barklin A. Systemic inflammation in the brain-dead organ donor. Acta Anaesthesiol Scand 2009;53:425–35.
56. Lansdale M, Gropper MA. Management of the potential organ donor in the ICU. ICU Dir 2012;3:185–8.
57. Bugge JF. Brain death and its implications for management of the potential organ donor. Acta Anaesthesiol Scand 2009;53:1239–50.

58. Kamarainen A, Virkkunen I, Tenhunen J. Hypothermic preconditioning of donor organs prior to harvesting and ischaemia using ice-cold intravenous fluids. Med Hypotheses 2009;73:65–6.
59. Novitzky D, Cooper DK. The brain-dead organ donor: pathophysiology and management. New York: Springer Science+Business Media; 2013.
60. Venkateswaran RV, Patchell VB, Wilson IC, et al. Early donor management increase the retrieval rate of lungs for transplantation. Ann Thorac Surg 2008; 85:278–86.
61. Al-Khafaji A, Murugan R, Wahed A, et al. Monitoring organ donors to improve transplantation results (MOnIToR) trial methodology. Crit Care Resusc 2013; 15:234–40.
62. Cantin B, Kwok BW, Chan MC, et al. The impact of brain death on survival after heart transplantation: time is of the essence. Transplantation 2003;76:1275–9.
63. Avlonitis VS, Fisher AJ, Kirby JA, et al. Pulmonary transplantation: the role of brain death in donor lung injury. Transplantation 2003;75:1928–33.
64. Wheeler AP, Bernard GR. Acute lung injury and the acute respiratory distress syndrome: a clinical review. Lancet 2007;369:1553–64.
65. Avlonitis VS, Wigfield CH, Kirby JA, et al. The hemodynamic mechanisms of lung injury and systemic inflammatory response following brain death in the transplant donor. Am J Transplant 2005;5:684–93.
66. Mascia L, Pasero D, Slutsky AS, et al. Effect of a lung protective strategy for organ donors on eligibility and availability of lungs for transplantation: a randomized controlled trial. JAMA 2010;304:2620–7.
67. Demetriades D, Lam L. Assessment, monitoring, and management of brain-dead potential organ donors in the USA. In: Novitzky D, Cooper DKC, editors. The brain-dead organ donor: pathophysiology and management. New York: Springer Science+Business Media; 2013. p. 209–16.
68. Curtis JR, Patrick D, Shannon S, et al. The family conference as a focus to improve communication about end-of-life care in the intensive care unit: opportunities for improvement. Crit Care Med 2001;29:N26–33.
69. Franz HG, DeJong W, Wolfe SM, et al. Explaining brain death: a critical feature of the donation process. Journal of Transplant Coordination: official publication of the North American Transplant Coordinators Organization (NATCO) 1997;7: 14–21.
70. Tawil I, Brown LH, Comfort D, et al. Family presence during brain death evaluation: a randomized controlled trial. Crit Care Med 2014;42:934–44.
71. Greer DM, Curiale GG. End-of-life and brain death in acute coma and disorders of consciousness. Semin Neurol 2013;33:157–66.
72. Bernat JL. Philosophical and ethical aspects of brain death. In: Wijdicks EFM, editor. Brain death. Philadelphia: Lippincott Williams & Wilkins; 2001. p. 171–87.

Index

Note: Page numbers of article titles are in **boldface** type.

Crit Care Clin 30 (2014) 833–841
http://dx.doi.org/10.1016/S0749-0704(14)00071-2
0749-0704/14/$ – see front matter © 2014 Elsevier Inc. All rights reserved.

criticalcare.theclinics.com

United States Postal Service

Statement of Ownership, Management, and Circulation
(All Periodicals Publications Except Requestor Publications)

1. Publication Title
Critical Care Clinics

2. Publication Number
0 0 0 - 7 0 8

3. Filing Date
9/1/4/14

4. Issue Frequency
Jan, Apr, Jul, Oct

5. Number of Issues Published Annually
4

6. Annual Subscription Price
$210.00

7. Complete Mailing Address of Known Office of Publication *(Not printer) (Street, city, county, state, and ZIP+4®)*

Elsevier Inc.
360 Park Avenue South
New York, NY 10010-1710

Contact Person
Stephen R. Bushing

Telephone *(Include area code)*
215-239-3688

8. Complete Mailing Address of Headquarters or General Business Office of Publisher *(Not printer)*

Elsevier Inc., 360 Park Avenue South, New York, NY 10010-1710

9. Full Names and Complete Mailing Addresses of Publisher, Editor, and Managing Editor *(Do not leave blank)*

Publisher *(Name and complete mailing address)*
Linda Belfus, Elsevier Inc., 1600 John F. Kennedy Blvd., Suite 1800, Philadelphia, PA 19103-2899

Editor *(Name and complete mailing address)*
Patrick Manley, Elsevier Inc., 1600 John F. Kennedy Blvd., Suite 1800, Philadelphia, PA 19103-2899

Managing Editor *(Name and complete mailing address)*
Adrianne Brigido, Elsevier Inc., 1600 John F. Kennedy Blvd., Suite 1800, Philadelphia, PA 19103-2899

10. Owner *(Do not leave blank. If the publication is owned by a corporation, give the name and address of the corporation immediately followed by the names and addresses of all stockholders owning or holding 1 percent or more of the total amount of stock. If not owned by a corporation, give the names and addresses of the individual owners. If owned by a partnership or other unincorporated firm, give its name and address as well as those of each individual owner. If the publication is published by a nonprofit organization, give its name and address.)*

Full Name	Complete Mailing Address
Wholly owned subsidiary of	1600 John F. Kennedy Blvd, Ste. 1800
Reed/Elsevier, US holdings	Philadelphia, PA 19103-2899

11. Known Bondholders, Mortgagees, and Other Security Holders Owning or Holding 1 Percent or More of Total Amount of Bonds, Mortgages, or Other Securities. If none, check box ☐ None

Full Name	Complete Mailing Address
N/A	

12. Tax Status *(For completion by nonprofit organizations authorized to mail at nonprofit rates)* (Check one)
The purpose, function, and nonprofit status of this organization and the exempt status for federal income tax purposes:
☐ Has Not Changed During Preceding 12 Months
☐ Has Changed During Preceding 12 Months *(Publisher must submit explanation of change with this statement)*

PS Form 3526, August 2012 (Page 1 of 3 (Instructions Page 3)) PSN 7530-01-000-9931 **PRIVACY NOTICE**: See our Privacy policy in www.usps.com

---

13. Publication Title
Critical Care Clinics

14. Issue Date for Circulation Data Below
April 2014

15. Extent and Nature of Circulation

			Average No. Copies Each Issue During Preceding 12 Months	No. Copies of Single Issue Published Nearest to Filing Date
a. Total Number of Copies *(Net press run)*			929	898
b. Paid Circulation (By Mail and Outside the Mail)	(1)	Mailed Outside-County Paid Subscriptions Stated on PS Form 3541. *(Include paid distribution above nominal rate, advertiser's proof copies, and exchange copies)*	540	520
	(2)	Mailed In-County Paid Subscriptions Stated on PS Form 3541 *(Include paid distribution above nominal rate, advertiser's proof copies, and exchange copies)*		
	(3)	Paid Distribution Outside the Mails Including Sales Through Dealers and Carriers, Street Vendors, Counter Sales, and Other Paid Distribution Outside USPS®	147	122
	(4)	Paid Distribution by Other Classes Mailed Through the USPS (e.g. First-Class Mail®)		
c. Total Paid Distribution *(Sum of 15b (1), (2), (3), and (4))*			687	642
d. Free or Nominal Rate Distribution (By Mail and Outside the Mail)	(1)	Free or Nominal Rate Outside-County Copies Included on PS Form 3541	69	71
	(2)	Free or Nominal Rate In-County Copies Included on PS Form 3541		
	(3)	Free or Nominal Rate Copies Mailed at Other Classes Through the USPS (e.g. First-Class Mail)		
	(4)	Free or Nominal Rate Distribution Outside the Mail (Carriers or other means)		
e. Total Free or Nominal Rate Distribution *(Sum of 15d (1), (2), (3) and (4))*			69	71
f. Total Distribution *(Sum of 15c and 15e)*			756	713
g. Copies not Distributed *(See instructions to publishers #4 (page #3))*			173	185
h. Total *(Sum of 15f and g)*			929	898
i. Percent Paid *(15c divided by 15f times 100)*			90.87%	90.04%

16. Total circulation includes electronic copies. Report circulation on PS Form 3526-X worksheet.

17. Publication of Statement of Ownership
☐ If the publication is a general publication, publication of this statement is required. Will be printed in the **October 2014** issue of this publication.

18. Signature and Title of Editor, Publisher, Business Manager, or Owner

[signature]

Stephen R. Bushing – Inventory Distribution Coordinator

Date
September 14, 2014

I certify that all information furnished on this form is true and complete. I understand that anyone who furnishes false or misleading information on this form or who omits material or information requested on the form may be subject to criminal sanctions (including fines and imprisonment) and/or civil sanctions (including civil penalties).

PS Form 3526, August 2012 (Page 2 of 3)

Printed and bound by CPI Group (UK) Ltd, Croydon, CR0 4YY

03/10/2024

01040495-0017